CW00972811

The Rainbow of De

Augusto Boal is one of the world's leading theatre practitioners; he is the inventor of a whole school of theatre, the Theatre of the Oppressed. Up to now, the Theatre of the Oppressed has concentrated on using theatre in political contexts, as a tool for understanding, education and development. His previous book, *Games for Actors and Non-Actors*, has been translated into numerous languages and is now a standard text for theatre people and those who work with communities. This book represents a new departure, showing as it does how theatre can be used in a therapeutic context to enhance personal and group development.

The Rainbow of Desire deals with four main areas: the theory behind the work; description of the techniques used, under two headings, 'prospective' and 'introspective'; and description of the work in practice. There is also an introduction by the translator, Adrian Jackson, and an afterpiece by Boal relating his most recent experiences using this work in India.

The originality of *The Rainbow of Desire* lies in its use of images as the main vocabulary for a psycho-therapeutic investigation. Rather than seeking to recreate past events, it works essentially in the here and now; it works with the reality of the image, rather than the image of reality. A bold and brilliant book, *The Rainbow of Desire* will make fascinating reading for anyone studying or making theatre or involved in therapy.

Augusto Boal is Vereador (Member of Parliament) of Rio de Janeiro and President of the Theatre of the Oppressed in Rio de Janeiro and Paris. Previous publications include *Games for Actors and Non-Actors* and *Theatre of the Oppressed*, both of which have been translated into numerous languages.

Adrian Jackson is Associate Director of the London Bubble Theatre and is also a freelance director and teacher. He was the translator of *Games for Actors and Non-Actors* into the English language (Routledge 1992).

The Rainbow of Desire

The Boal Method of Theatre and Therapy

Augusto Boal

Translated by Adrian Jackson

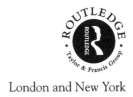

London and New York

First published 1995
by Routledge
11 New Fetter Lane, London EC4P 4EE

Simultaneously published in the USA and Canada
by Routledge
29 West 35th Street, New York, NY 10001

Reprinted 1996, 1998, 1999

Routledge is an imprint of the Taylor & Francis Group

Original text © 1995 Augusto Boal
Introduction and translation © 1995 Adrian Jackson

Typeset in Monotype Janson by
J&L Composition Ltd, Filey, North Yorkshire
Printed and bound in Great Britain by
T.J. International Ltd, Padstow, Cornwall
Text design: Simon Josebury

British Library Cataloguing in Publication Data
A catalogue record for this book is available from the British Library

Library of Congress Cataloging in Publication Data
A catalog record for this book is available from the Library of Congress

ISBN 0–415–10349–5

For Lula,
for Paulo Freire,
for the Workers'
Party of Brazil

For Groto Loutz
and
Zerka Moreno

Contents

CONTENTS

TRANSLATOR'S INTRODUCTION

The trajectory of Augusto Boal's work can be mapped as a series of epiphanies, a series of discoveries, a continuous process of response to his own perception of the inadequacy of what he was doing before; this is a very self-critical work, which thrives on problems. Viewed over its forty-year history, the work glides naturally, organically, from the socio-political to the socio-individual to the individual-political and back again – but it is always rooted in practice, and it is always theatre. The main body of theory, as articulated in 'The Theatre of the Oppressed' has stood the test of time, and is constantly refreshed and invigorated by the energetic, urgent extension and development of practice.

This book represents the latest staging point in this journey, the exposition of 'The Rainbow of Desire', the name Boal gives to a collection of theatrical techniques and exercises designed to harness the power of 'the aesthetic space' (the stage) to examine individual, internalised oppressions and to place them within a larger context. But this is by no means the last word in the Theatre of the Oppressed – at the time of writing, Boal is already surging forward with his next project, the Legislative Theatre, a way of using theatre within a political system to produce a truer form of democracy.

For every development in Boalian practice, there is a story; in his introduction, he tells us the story of Virgilio, which exposed the inadequacy of the brand of agit-prop theatre Boal was involved in at the time – or rather its inadequacy for that particular moment. In the aftermath of Virgilio comes the invention/discovery of simultaneous dramaturgy, in which actors present a problem, audiences suggest solutions and the actors then enact them; till that too runs up against an obstacle, in the next story – the formidable figure of the woman who feels the actors are not accurately enacting her 'idea' and invades the stage to show it herself – and Forum Theatre is born. In Forum, the audience not only comments on the action, it intervenes directly in the action, taking the protagonist's part and trying to bring the play to a different end; it is no longer a passive receiver, it is a gathering of 'spect-actors' (active spectators) who bring their own experience and suggestions to the question, 'What is to be done ?'

The Cop in the Head/Rainbow of Desire techniques are also a

response to experimental practice; these are not supported by a single story but by a repeated perception, during a period of European and North American exile from Brazil, that participants in Boal's Forum Theatre workshops were frequently asking if the work could deal with oppressions where there was no visible, tangible, present oppressor. As ably anatomised by Mady Schutzman and Jan Cohen-Cruz in *Playing Boal*,◉ Boal's transplantation to the West brought him into contact, particularly in his workshops, with people who found it less easy than peasant and worker groups he had worked with in Brazil and other Latin American countries, to synthesise their experience of the world into the sort of Manichaean equation suggested by the terms 'oppressor' and 'oppressed'; this confrontation – and the resulting proposition by groups of 'emptiness', 'fear' and the like as fit 'oppressions' to treat with this work – led directly to the invention or discovery of the Cop in the Head/Rainbow of Desire techniques.

◉ *Playing Boal*, ed. M. Schutzman and J. Cohen-Cruz, London: Routledge, 1994.

This rewriting of techniques is a cumulative process, an aggregation not a cancelling out; Boal still respects and uses all the earlier techniques (agit-prop, invisible theatre, forum theatre etc.) in situations to which they are applicable. Forum Theatre is the foundation-stone for the new, as yet underdeveloped Legislative Theatre; as a newly elected member of the Rio Chamber of Vereadores (like a very important City Council), for the PT, the Workers' Party, Boal is using Forum as a tool for communities to suggest laws they would like to see enacted, which his theatre groups then take back to a lawyer to be drafted into formal laws; Boal then puts these laws forward in the Chamber to be voted on. Forum Theatre and Image Theatre techniques both have a central place in this new psycho-therapeutic arena.

Actually of course, Forum was never about a simplification into right and wrong, never in absolute terms of black and white – one person's black might be another's white, or grey, or red, or blue or yellow, or whatever. Forum is always about what a roomful of people believe at a particular moment in time, and what one roomful of people believe is not necessarily the same as what the next roomful will believe. Forum never seeks to impose any kind of doctrine of political correctness, nor to make things easy; easier to understand, maybe. The joker's function is not that of facilitator, the joker is (in Boal-speak) a 'difficultator', undermining easy judgements, reinforcing our grasp of the complexity of a situation, but not letting that complexity get in the way of action or frighten us into submission or inactivity. Things aren't always what they seem, it says; let's try and do something about them.

This fascination with problematising is an ongoing feature, which overlaps from Forum into Rainbow; looking at the problem is at least as important as finding solutions. Looking at the problem is in itself therapeutic: it is a step toward doing something about it. A therapy which continually throws light on problems, a variety of different shades of light, is by definition more dynamic than one which seeks (and stops at) a solution. Which is not to say that, in both kinds of work, concrete, workable solutions do not frequently arise – they do, but we need not stop there.

In the Rainbow of Desire as in Forum Theatre work, we work on the case of an individual, and from that individual case we extrapolate into the group present, and then, sometimes, from that group into the larger society of which it is a microcosm or a fragment. This process Boal calls 'ascesis', the movement from the phenomenon to the law which regulates phenomena of that kind; and his concept of 'osmosis' enables this free play from one arena to the other, suggesting as it does that no individual consciousness can remain unmarked by societal values. There are cops in our head, they must have come from somewhere – and if they are in our head, maybe they are in other people's heads as well. Where did they come from and what are we going to do about them ?

The basic vocabulary of the Rainbow of Desire work is Image Theatre. In almost all cases, the techniques start with an improvisation based on an actual situation, which is initially cast and directed by its real-life protagonist, who plays him- or herself. This is then used as a launch-pad for the investigation – the improvisation, not the original event; in most of the techniques, there is no requirement for the protagonist ever to explain the original story to more than a couple of people. Images of the characters 'present' in the improvisation, seen or unseen but detected, are made and offered by both the protagonists and the larger group of spectators present. These images are then 'dynamised' in various ways, to bring them to life, and the results are observed, objectively. Both objective and subjective commentaries are invited, as long as they are clearly defined in either category. Here there are no misreadings, only multiple readings, and the readings most wildly at odds with each other are often the most fruitful and revealing. The observations are collated, discussed and relayed back to the protagonist. Any 'conclusions' arrived at are strictly subjective, and classified as such, and it is up to the protagonist to make of them what he or she will.

An ossified, unreconstructed Marxist reading of Boal's movement in the therapeutic arena might be that it is a relapse into bourgeois individualism; this is as unhelpful as it is facile. The truth of the matter is that the work to date has always had therapeutic effects, and that these effects have been as much on individuals as societies. Therapeutic is not necessarily a synonym for normalising or societising.

As Daniel Feldhendler has observed[©], there has been a movement in Boal's thinking on 'catharsis', an acceptance that the Aristotelian (and in Boal's terms coercive) definition of catharsis need not be the sole working definition of the word. If, in *The Theatre of the Oppressed* (London: pub. Pluto Press, 1979), Boal interpreted Aristotelian catharsis as a purging by society of its members' asocial tendencies, the Boalian redefinition in this book suggests that individuals, and by extension society itself, can be changed by a catharsis, that catharsis is not the sole province of the controlling group; that it is a weapon that can be pointed in either direction. His catharsis is a removal of blocks, not a voiding of desires; the desires are clarified and dynamised, not tamed. Here catharsis releases desires which societal constructions (such as family, school or work) had imprisoned. Individuals can be neurotic – perhaps whole societies, nations even, can be neurotic – and perhaps there is a connection between the two phenomena; see the story of the captain in the mirror, p. 99 ff.

If there is a story which goes with this development of the Theatre of the Oppressed, it may be Boal's beautiful Brechtian parable, 'The Political Master Swimmer.'[©] In this story the eponymous swimmer hesitates and then refuses to rescue a drowning man, with the words,

> 'Excuse me, dear Sir, but I am a political Master Swimmer and you are nothing but a single individual. When there are at least twenty of you drowning together, then I will be at your service, ready to help you and save your life.'

This counterblast to accusations of bourgeois individualism amply demonstrates Boal's dissatisfaction with dogma, his essential allegiance to humanity. As he says in this book, 'if I can help, I do'. He cares about people before ideas, which is why he will always be a man of the theatre whose work is political, rather than a politician who works with theatre.

© Daniel Feldhendler, 'Augusto Boal and Jacob Moreno: Theatre and Therapy', in *Playing Boal*.

© In *Playing Boal*.

In any case, Boal himself makes clear that, far from this work being a luxury to be enjoyed only by the economically privileged West, his Brazilian groups and others as far afield as Calcutta have a hunger to do it. The implantation of oppression in our heads is not nullified because we face concrete 'actual' oppressions outside – far from it: the two work inextricably together, they compound each other. My own work with homeless people has quickly brought me to the realisation that though many of the roots of their problems are economic, the solutions must involve a far broader panoply of disciplines if they are to stand any chance of being successful. We have used many of these techniques with some success.

At the risk of apparent deviation, one could also refer such hardened critics to Beckett – apropos of Susan Sontag's production of *Waiting for Godot* in a besieged Sarajevo: how could this pinnacle of modernism perform a useful function in a war-torn, besieged city, struggling daily, hour to hour, for its basic human necessities, its citizens scavenging like animals to survive? The answer lies in the question – we are *more* than animals, we need more than bread. In Sarajevo, Beckett's play is revealed as the simple parable it is, and performs the same function of reflecting, symbolising, clarifying as all good theatre always does. Extraordinary to think of the puzzlement the play met with on its first outing, the incomprehension of a play as transparent as Adam and Eve – not a creation myth but a survival myth. Equally extraordinary the amazement that productions in San Quentin jail or Sarajevo should find some resonance. Boal's work, in as extreme if not as sensational contexts, similarly places theatre at the centre of human life, 'a vocation for all humanity'.

In the Rainbow of Desires there is another continuity with the preceding work, which is located in Boal's desire to democratise, to demystify, processes which have become the sole province of 'professionals'. Having democratised theatre, now he works on democratising therapy (and next he is working on democratising politics, the largest undertaking yet!). If everyone can and does act, as demonstrated by Forum Theatre which relieves audiences of the obligation to be passive, perhaps everyone can also play a part in the therapeutic process – and perhaps they can play the largest part themselves. Here the 'patient' is not a passive recipient of treatment, but, like the film-director inmates of Sartrouville (p. 47), is the director of his or her own therapeutic process, with the presence of a participating audience acting as a multiple mirror to enable new and multiple readings of past (and always present) events.

Present to future is the dynamic Boal works along – if the work involves reminiscence it is not with a view to the past's preservation in aspic, but to a rewriting of the present which has been coloured by that past. When a participant tells a story from their past, we concentrate on their telling and their presentation of that story, here and now, in the present; we observe and comment on what we are witnessing, which we know is happening, not what happened in the past, which we only have one person's word for.

Just as with the foregoing work, these techniques can be practised by any group. They need a certain amount of preparation, and it is preferable if the group has been working together for some length of time. Beyond that, the only skills necessary are observation and openness. Two words recur, with particular usages, in this book – surprise and admiration (the latter in its original sense of wondering at, standing back from something in astonishment). These two words, describing qualities which may need nurture in a weary and knowledgeable world, describe qualities Boal himself displays in abundance; read the afterpiece to this book, revealing his wonder at the state of affairs he meets in India. Surprise is in itself a rebellion; it says, 'No, I do not accept this as normal'; 'Whose "normal"?' 'Why is this called normal?' Admiration, as Boal uses it, brings with it a sense of discovery, which helps consolidate what is learnt in the theatrical process.

There is one important note to be observed on the use of this book, which has to do with rules and rituals: in essence it is that this book is not a rule-book, the processes are not to be followed slavishly. The techniques should be adapted to suit the participants, not vice versa. Boal's entire theatrical career is based on the disruption and subversion of theatrical ritual, even his own invented rituals. We saw this towards the end of a Festival of the Theatre of the Oppressed in Rio in 1993 when a flawed piece of Forum Theatre dealing with AIDS was presented and promptly disrupted by angry spect-actors, and a by this time quite tired Boal came on from the sidelines invigorated and fascinated to understand and deal with this anger. Many times in this book he refers to the breaking of rules newly established, without fear, with relish – what will we find out if we do it this way?

There may be some comparative exceptions to this – Forum Theatre has a few givens which have really stood the test of time, and in a sense it is time-wasting to try them out again – but if that is what the audience needs, that is what they need. Boal's pedagogy never delivers the finished article to its audience to be digested whole – if anything it delivers a process, a provocation. The rules in this book should be treated with a similar combination of respect and disrespect – like a good cook, users of the book should be prepared to vary the recipe to suit the ingredients and the tastes of the eaters, because the work is always about what is going on in the moment, not what is going on on the page. It is not a catechism.

All this begs the question of what the work actually does, what its effects are on individuals or groups. I can only answer partially, from observation of participants in Boal's and my own workshops. As far as I know, no one has yet attempted any follow-up study after a workshop: such an initiative would probably be doomed to failure, as we are often dealing with unquantifiable changes which resist statistical analysis; the observable changes are qualitative.

Participation in this work seems to bring with it some ease, in the context of a dissatisfaction. Like the whole of the Theatre of the Oppressed, it thrives on dissatisfaction: implicitly it says, do not be satisfied with less than you need; are you satisfied? If not, why not? If you're not happy, let's do something about it. Its essential declared goal is happiness, but not happiness as a static condition, a laid-back nirvana, happiness as a busyness, an aliveness, a full capacity, a firing on all cylinders. When it is working, people often seem to leave the workshops with a clarity and a sense of determination to sort things out; and not only the protagonists, because, though the work is centred on the teller of a story, the story is populated by other members of the group who are grappling with their own analogous problems.

There are other benefits from this work and other usages. For groups which have problems of internal dynamics or recurring misunderstanding, various of the exercises can be used to help analyse what is going wrong: exercises like Rashomon, The Image of the Group, and so on. The basic image work is what lends the techniques their theatricality – because of the extremity of the images, their rigidity, and the frequently anti-naturalistic dynamisations of them, the techniques often yield up better theatre than conventional naturalistic psychodrama. This same theatricality can equally be put at the service of the rehearsal process for a 'normal' play; a number of directors in 'mainstream' theatres, including myself, are already using the work in this way. Taking the work even further from its original intention, but with interesting results, writers' groups are using the techniques to study and develop their fictional characters.

Sometimes participants from a psycho-therapeutic training background express worries about 'closure': is it safe to let people go off with so many thoughts buzzing in their heads? Do we need to calm everybody down? Should we have a massed hug by way of ending? My experience is that usually if the group needs such forms of closure, they will do it themselves or ask for it; occasionally, one can see that someone is not being provided for by the group, in which case the director of the session should take action. But, on the whole, people only bring what they want to bring to such a workshop: no one is obliged to say anything more, or go any further, than they want. People certainly leave with things to do, the job is only started, there is no doubt about that – but that is as it should be. Being over-protective can be patronising.

Two small translation notes. I have used he and she in roughly equal quantities I hope, where gender was not relevant and where pluralising would have led to complication. Three French words – *personne, personnalité,* and *personnage* – work so well as a triad that I have not translated the third, *personnage,* which means character, as in a play; *dramatis persona* is close, but cumbersome.

At the time of writing, Boal is preparing for the Workers' Party (PT) campaign for the general election – a clear signal, if any were needed, that he has lost none of his political fervour and none of his anger against social injustice. The odds are stacked massively against his party, in a country where television is a virtual private monopoly in very reactionary hands. But let us hope the PT are successful; apart from anything else, it would be wonderful to see the effects of his Legislative Theatre experiment were his party in power. His own campaigning logo, when he was seeking election to the Chamber of Vereadores, improbably enough bore the phrase 'Coragem de ser feliz' – 'Have the courage to be happy.' His optimism and faith in humanity are indefatigable.

By way of conclusion it might seem improbable to quote Chekhov in the context of Boal (though I must admit to having always secretly longed for the Forum Theatre version of *The Three Sisters* – let's vote on whether you should go to Moscow or not, perhaps you should go for a couple of days and see if you like it, perhaps you should all seek some sort of family therapy because going to Moscow is actually only masking other desires and frustrations – the possibilities are endless). But when asked what the message of his plays was, Chekhov famously answered: 'You cannot live like this . . . ' Maybe Boal might add, 'unless you're sure you want to'.

Adrian Jackson
March 1994

WHY THIS BOOK? MY THREE
THEATRICAL ENCOUNTERS

A long journey has led me to this point. My fortieth year of working in theatre approaches. And still I have many things left to do – some already conceived, yet to be executed, others as yet unconceived, but already prefigured. This book marks a new stage, the end of a long period of research. This is still the Theatre of the Oppressed, but a new Theatre of the Oppressed. How did I get here?

At the start of the 1960s I travelled extensively with my theatre company – the Teatro de Arena de São Paulo (the Arena Theatre of São Paulo). We went into poor areas, to some of the most poverty-stricken parts of Brazil: the interior of São Paulo, the North-East. . . . Extreme poverty is still an abiding feature in Brazil. Suffice it to say that the average monthly wage is less than 50 US dollars and most of the population doesn't earn even that. According to recent, reliable surveys, a middle-ranking worker today takes home less than the minimum spent by a master in the last century to feed, clothe and tend his slave. Yet Brazil ranks eighth in the league of international capitalist economies. Extreme opulence exists alongside the most abject misery there. And as idealistic artists, we could not be accomplices to such cruelty. We rebelled against it, our blood boiled, we suffered. We wrote and staged plays, spirited, violent pieces, aggressive in their anger against injustice. We were heroic in our writing of them, sublime in our performance: almost always these plays would end with anthems of exhortation, sung in chorus by the actors, with verses which urged: Let us spill our blood for freedom! Let us spill our blood for our land! Let us spill our blood, let us spill our blood!

It seemed right to us, indeed a matter of great urgency, to exhort the oppressed to struggle against oppression. Which oppressed? All of them. The oppressed in a general sense. Too general a sense. And we made use of our art to tell Truths, to bring Solutions. We taught the peasants how to fight for their lands – we, who lived in the big cities. We taught the blacks how to combat racial prejudice – we, who were almost all very, very white. We taught women how to struggle against their oppressors. Which oppressors? Why, us, since we were feminists to a man – and virtually all of us were men. Nevertheless, the intention was good.

But one day – in every story one day comes along sooner or later – so, one fine day, we were performing one of these splendid musical plays for an audience of peasants in a small village in the North-East – and we sang the heroic text 'Let us spill our blood!', to our rapt audience made up only of peasants. At the end of the show a huge peasant, a great big strapping colossus of a man, came up to us, on the verge of tears:

> 'Here's a fine thing – people like you, young people, town people, who think exactly like us. We're right with you, we also think we must give our blood for our land.'

We were proud. Mission accomplished. Our message had been received loud and clear. But Virgilio – I will never forget his name, his face, his silent tears – Virgilio went on:

> 'Since you think exactly like us, this is what we're going to do: we'll have lunch [it was midday], and afterwards we'll all go together, you with your guns, we with ours, and send the colonel's[◉] bullyboys packing – they've taken over a comrade's land, set fire to his house and threatened to kill his family – But first, let's eat . . . .'

⊙ In Brazil, big landowners call themselves 'colonel', which designation has however no military significance. In the same way, in large towns, industrialists and big businessmen call themselves 'doctor', without necessarily having any connection whatsoever with medicine or any other academic discipline.

We had lost our appetite.

Trying to match our thoughts with our words, we did our best to clear up the misunderstanding. Honesty seemed the best policy: our guns were theatrical props, they were not real weapons.

> 'Guns which don't fire?' Virgilio asked, in astonishment. 'Then, what are they for?'

> 'They are for doing plays, they can't actually be fired. We are serious artists, we believe in what we preach, we are quite genuine, but the guns are . . . fakes.'

> 'OK, since the guns are fakes, let's chuck them. But you people aren't fakes, you're genuine, I saw you singing about how blood must be spilt, I was there. You are genuine, so come with us, we have guns enough for everyone.'

Our fear turned to panic. Because it was difficult to explain – both to Virgilio and to ourselves – how we could be sincere and genuine and true even though our guns wouldn't fire and we didn't know how to shoot. We explained ourselves as best we could. If we agreed to go with them, we would be more of a hindrance than a help.

'So, when you *true artists* talk of the blood that must be spilt, this blood you sing about spilling – it's our blood you mean, not yours, isn't that so?'

'We are true to the cause, absolutely, but we are true artists not true peasants! Virgilio, come back, let's talk about it. . . . Come back.'

I never saw him again.

I have not forgotten Virgilio. Nor have I forgotten that moment, a moment when I felt ashamed of my art – which, in itself, still seemed a fine thing to me. Where was the error? Certainly not in the theatrical genre, which, even to this day, I believe to be justified. Agit-prop – agitation and propaganda – can be an extremely effective instrument in political struggle. The error lay in the use to which we put it.

Around that time, Che Guevara wrote a very beautiful phrase: *solidarity means running the same risks.* This helped us understand our error. Agit-prop is fine; what was not fine was that we were incapable of following our own advice. We white men from the big city, there was very little we could teach black women of the country. . . .

Since that first encounter – an encounter with a real peasant, in flesh and blood, rather than an abstract 'peasantry' – an encounter which traumatised but enlightened, I have never again written plays that give advice, nor have I ever sent "messages" again. Except on occasions when I was running the same risks as everyone else.

In Peru, where I worked in 1973 within the framework of a theatre-based literacy project, I began to use a new form of theatre, which I named *simultaneous dramaturgy*. Simultaneous dramaturgy consisted of this: we would present a play that chronicled a problem to which we wanted to find a solution. The play would run its course up to the moment of crisis – the crucial point at which the protagonist had to make a decision. At this point, we would stop performing and ask the audience what the protagonist should do. Everyone would make their own suggestions. And on stage the performers would improvise each of these suggestions, till all had been exhausted.

This was already progress. We were no longer giving advice, we were learning together. But the actors still retained their 'power', their dominion of the stage. The suggestions came from the audience, sure, but on stage it was still we, the artists, who interpreted what had been suggested.

This theatrical form was a great success. But one fine day, a shy woman came to see me. She said:

> 'I know that you do political theatre, and my problem is not political, but it is a very big problem and it's mine. Perhaps you could help me with your theatre?'

I told her that, in my opinion, all problems are political, but she replied that this was not so in her case. Why? Because, she said, her problem was her husband. 'You see – you said "my husband", and who tells you that that man is your husband? Society married you to him, so your problem is political . . . .'

For myself, if I am able to help other people, then I do so. She told me her story: every month, sometimes several times a month, her husband used to ask her for money to pay the monthly instalments on the house which – he said – he was having built for them. The husband, who only did odd jobs here and there, earned very little. Anyway, she used to hand over their savings to him. From time to time he would give her 'receipts' in exchange for the monthly payments, receipts which were handwritten and scented. When she asked to see the house, he would reply: 'Later.' But she never got to see anything. And she began to have doubts. One day, they had an argument. So she decided to call her neighbour – who could read – and ask her to read the perfumed receipts. They were not receipts; they were love letters, sent by the husband's lover and carefully stored in the mattress by his illiterate wife.

> 'My husband has gone away – he said he was working all week in Chaclacayo as a mason. But now it's obvious where he's really gone. He comes back tomorrow. What am I to do?'

> 'I don't know, madam. Let us ask the people.'

Maybe it was not so political, but it was certainly a big problem. We decided to accept her proposition and that very evening, having constructed a scenario, we enacted the play using the 'simultaneous dramaturgy' mode. Come the moment of crisis – the husband rings the doorbell – what to do? I myself had no idea, I appealed to the audience for ideas. Solutions came pouring in:

'This is what she should do: let him in, tell him that she has found out the truth and start to cry, really cry, cry for a good twenty minutes. Then he will feel guilty, he will repent, and she can forgive him. You know ... for a woman to be on her own in this country is very dangerous. ...'

We improvised the solution and the tears. Repentance came, followed by forgiveness, but followed also by the dissatisfaction of a second woman spectator.

'No, that's all wrong! What she should do is lock the husband out!'

We improvised the lockout. The actor husband, a very thin young man, was delighted:

'Oh yeah? Great! Today was payday, I'll take my wages to my lover, and I'll go and live with her.'

A third woman proposed the opposite solution: the wife should leave the husband all alone in the house, abandon him for good. The husband-actor was even more delighted: he immediately brought his lover over to the house to live with him.

Suggestions continued to rain down. We improvised them all. Suddenly I became aware of a very large, powerful woman – built like one of those Japanese 'sumo' fighters – seated in the third row, shaking her head vigorously and almost bursting with rage. I was afraid, because she seemed to be glaring at me with a look of absolute hatred. As gently as possible, I said:

'Madam, I get the feeling that you might have an idea. Tell us and we'll improvise it.'

'This is what she should do: let the husband in, have a clear conversation with him, and then, and only then, forgive him.'

I was completely baffled. With all her huffing and puffing, and muttered comments, and looks that could kill, I was expecting her to propose solutions of a more violent nature. Anyway, I didn't argue, and I told the actors to improvise this new solution. They improvised, but without any real gusto. The husband protested his love and – all's well that ends well – asked his wife to bring him his supper. She went off to the kitchen and that's how the scene ended.

I looked at the big woman; she was huffing and puffing more than ever and her fulminating glare was even more furious and murderous than before.

'Madam, I am terribly sorry, but we have done what you suggested: the woman had a clear talk with her husband, and afterwards she forgave him. And it looks like from now on they can be happy.'

'But that's not what I said. I said that she should explain things to him clearly, very clearly, and that afterwards – and only afterwards – she could forgive him.'

'To my mind that is exactly what we have just improvised, but, if you like, we can do it again.'

'I do like. Do it!'

I then asked the actress to exaggerate a bit during her explanation, to explain as clearly as possible, and to extract the deepest, most sincere explanations from the husband. Which she and the actor-husband then did. Everything having been very well explained, the husband, now amorous and forgiven, asked his wife to go to the kitchen and get his supper. They were on the point of going off to live together happily ever after when I spotted the big woman, more furious, more threatening and more dangerous than ever. Somewhat nervous and, I'll admit, not a little frightened – I said to her:

'Madam, we are doing our best to try your suggestion, but you are never satisfied . . . .'

'No, you are not ! Because you are a man you don't want to try something a woman is telling you to do!'

'Madam, we are doing our best to understand what you want, we are trying to make the explanations as clear as we possibly can. If you are still not satisfied, why don't you come on stage yourself and show us what you mean by "a very clear conversation" – what is that?'

Illuminated, transfigured, the big woman took a deep breath, swelled once again to her full size and, eyes flashing, asked:

'May I?'

'You may!'

She came up on stage, grabbed the poor defenceless actor-husband (who was a real actor, but not a real husband, and moreover was skinny and weak), and laid into him with a broom-handle with all her strength, simultaneously delivering a lecture to him on her complete views on the relations between husband and wife. We attempted to rescue our endangered comrade, but the big woman was much stronger than us. Finally, she stopped of her own accord and, satisfied, planted her victim on a seat at the table and said:

> 'Now that we have had this very clear and very sincere conversation, *you* can go to the kitchen and fetch *my* dinner, because after all this I am tired out!'

As clarity goes, this was pretty clear. It could not have been clearer.

Even more clearly, this truth dawned on me: when the spectator herself comes on stage and carries out the action she has in mind, she does it in a manner which is personal, unique and non-transferable, as she alone can do it, and as no artist can do it in her place. On stage the actor is an interpreter who, in the act of translating, plays false. It is impossible not to play false. 'Tradutore, traditore', as the Italians have it.

This is how Forum Theatre was born. In this new kind of theatre, the debate does not come at the end – the forum is the show. Which is, in a manner of speaking, a desecration: we desecrate the stage, that altar over which usually the artist presides alone. We destroy the work offered by the artists in order to construct a new work out of it, together. A theatre which is not didactic, in the old sense of the word and style, but pedagogic, in the sense of a collective learning.

With Virgilio, I had learnt to see a human being, rather than simply a social class; the peasant rather than the peasantry, struggling with his social and political problems. With the big Peruvian woman, I learnt to see the human being struggling with her own problems, individual problems, which though they may not concern the totality of a class, nevertheless concern the totality of a life. And are no less important for that. But still to come was the lesson I was to learn during my European exile.

Living first in Lisbon, then in Paris, I worked for some fifteen years in various European countries, with immigrants, teachers, men and women, workers born in these countries, people who suffered oppressions with which I was well acquainted in Latin America: racism, sexism, intolerable working conditions, insufficient wages, police abuses of power, and so on. But in these

Theatre of the Oppressed workshops there also appeared oppressions which were new to me: 'loneliness', the 'impossibility of communicating with others', 'fear of emptiness'. For someone like me, fleeing explicit dictatorships of a cruel and brutal nature, it was natural that these themes should at first seem superficial and scarcely worthy of attention. It was as if I was always asking, mechanically: 'But where are the cops?' Because I was used to working with concrete, visible oppressions.

Little by little, I changed my opinion. I discovered, for instance, that the percentage of suicides was much higher in countries like Sweden or Finland – where the essential needs of the citizen in matters of housing, health, food and social security are met – than in countries like ours, Third World countries. In Latin America, the major killer is hunger; in Europe, it is drug overdose. But, whatever form it comes in, death is still death. And, thinking about the suffering of a person who chooses to take his or her own life in order to put an end to the fear of emptiness or the pangs of loneliness, I decided to work with these new oppressions and to consider them as such.

In Paris, at the beginning of the 1980s, I led a workshop which ran over a period of two years, *Flic dans la Tête* (The Cop in the Head). I started from the following hypothesis: the cops are in our heads, but their headquarters and barracks must be on the outside. The task was to discover how these 'cops' got into our heads, and to invent ways of dislodging them. It was an audacious proposition.

Throughout the last few years I have continued to work on this aspect of the Theatre of the Oppressed, this superposition of fields: the theatrical and the therapeutic. At the end of 1988 I was invited by Dr Grete Leutz, president of the International Association of Group Psychotherapists, to speak to the opening conference of the 10th world congress of this organisation, which took place in August and September 1989 in Amsterdam, on the centenary of the birth of Jacob L. Moreno, founder of the Association and inventer of psychodrama. I was also able to present to the psychotherapists participating in the congress – amongst whom was the widow of Jacob Moreno, Dr Zerka Moreno – the Rainbow of Desires technique. This invitation finally decided me to write this book, in which for the first time I set down a complete systematisation of all the techniques used in this research to date. Some are amply illustrated by cases which seemed to me exemplary; others – either because they are extremely clear or because they have already had exposure in my earlier books – are only described in their mode of functioning.

This book also contains a theoretical section, in which I try to explain the reason for the extraordinary power, the intense and effective energy, of the theatric event in domains outside the theatre: the political, the social, the fields of education and psychotherapy.

Part One | The Theory

1 THEATRE, THE FIRST HUMAN INVENTION

Theatre is the first human invention and also the invention which paves the way for all other inventions and discoveries.

Theatre is born when the human being discovers that it can observe itself; when it discovers that, in this act of seeing, it can see *itself* – see itself *in situ*: see itself seeing.

Observing itself, the human being perceives what it is, discovers what it is not and imagines what it could become. It perceives where it is and where it is not, and imagines where it could go. A triad comes into being. The observing-I, the I-*in-situ*, and the not-I, that is, the other. The human being alone possesses this faculty for self-observation in an imaginary mirror. (Doubtless it will have had prior experience of other mirrors – its mother's eyes, its reflection in water – but henceforward it is able to view itself by means of imagination alone.) The 'aesthetic space', which we will treat later, offers this imaginary mirror.

Therein resides the essence of theatre: in the human being observing itself. *The human being not only 'makes' theatre: it 'is' theatre.* And some human beings, besides being theatre, also make theatre. We all of us are; some of us also do.

Theatre has nothing to do with buildings or other physical constructions. Theatre – or theatricality – is this capacity, this human property which allows man to observe himself in action, in activity. The self-knowledge thus acquired allows him to be the subject (the one who observes) of another subject (the one who acts). It allows him to imagine variations of his action, to study alternatives. Man can see himself in the act of seeing, in the act of acting, in the act of feeling, the act of thinking. Feel himself feeling, think himself thinking.

The cat chases the rat, the lion pursues its prey, but neither animal is capable of self-observation. When a man hunts a bison, he sees himself in the act of hunting; which is why he can paint a picture of the hunter – himself – hunting the bison. He can invent painting because he has invented theatre: he has seen himself in the act of seeing. An actor, acting, taking action, he has learnt to be his own spectator. This spectator (spect-actor) is not only an object; he is a subject because he can also act on the actor – the spect-actor is the actor, he can guide him, change him. A spect-actor acting on the actor who acts.

Birds sing, but know nothing about music. Singing forms part of their animal activity – along with eating, drinking, coupling – and their song never varies; a nightingale will never try to sing like a swallow, nor a thrush like a lark. But the human being is capable of singing and seeing itself in the act of singing. That is why it can imitate animals, discover variations of its own song, compose. Birds are not composers, they are not even interpreters of music. They sing, just as they eat, drink and couple. Only the human being is tri-dimensional (the I who observes, the I-*in-situ* and the not-I) because it alone is capable of dichotomy (seeing itself seeing). And as it places itself inside and outside its situation, actually there, potentially here, it needs to symbolise that distance which separates space and divides time, the distance from 'I am' to 'I can be', and from present to future; it needs to symbolise this potential, to create symbols which occupy the space of *what is, but does not exist* concretely, of what is possible and could one day exist. So it creates symbolic languages: painting, music, words. Animals have access only to a language of signals (signs made up of calls, grunts, grimaces). The alarm call of an African monkey will be understood perfectly by an Amazonian monkey of the same species,[◉] but the word signifying alarm – *danger* – spoken in good Portuguese, will never be understood by a Swede or a Norwegian (who will, however, be able to understand the alarm signalled by the face of the person calling).

◉ We know that some big monkeys have a tribal language: they make specific references to 'this tree' or 'that tree'. But it remains a signaletic language; they are capable of talking about the danger of this tree (signal), but incapable of understanding the concept of tree (symbol).

The being becomes human when it invents theatre.

In the beginning, actor and spectator coexisted in the same person; the point at which they were separated, when some specialised as actors and others as spectators, marks the birth of the theatrical forms we know today. Also born at this time were 'theatres', architectural constructions intended to make sacred this division, this specialisation. The profession of 'actor' takes its first bow.

The theatrical profession, which belongs to a few, should not hide the existence and permanence of the theatrical vocation, which belongs to all. Theatre is a vocation for all human beings: it is the true nature of humanity.

The Theatre of the Oppressed is a system of physical exercises, aesthetic games, image techniques and special improvisations whose goal is to safeguard, develop and reshape this human vocation, by turning the practice of theatre into an effective tool for the comprehension of social and personal problems and the search for their solutions.

The Theatre of the Oppressed has three main branches – the educational, the social and the therapeutic. This book, which is focused on the therapeutic branch, uses old techniques from the 'arsenal'[⊙] of the Theatre of the Oppressed in new ways, and introduces recent techniques (1988–93) specific to the Cop in the Head. I hope that they will be as useful in the field of therapy as in the domain of theatre. (At the present moment, in Brazil, having recently been elected 'Vereador' (city councillor) for Rio de Janeiro, I am trying to develop a new possible application of Theatre of the Oppressed, the 'Legislative Theatre'. But it is still in its beginnings. . . .)

The title 'The Rainbow of Desire' is inspired by the name of one technique presented here. In fact, all the techniques have something to do with the rainbow of desire: all try to assist the analysis of its colours, with a view to combining them in other desired proportions, configurations and frameworks.

⊙ The name given to the entire organised ensemble of exercises, games and techniques of the Theatre of the Oppressed.

2 HUMAN BEINGS, A PASSION AND A PLATFORM: THE 'AESTHETIC SPACE'

What is theatre?

Over the centuries theatre has been defined in thousands of ways. Of these definitions, to my mind the simplest and most essential is that provided by Lope de Vega, for whom 'theatre is two human beings, a passion and a platform'. Theatre is the *passionate combat* of *two human beings* on *a platform*.

Two beings – not just one – because theatre studies the multiple interrelations of men and women living in society, rather than limiting itself to the contemplation of each solitary individual taken in isolation. Theatre denotes conflict, contradiction, confrontation, defiance. And the dramatic action lies in the variation and movement of this equation, of these opposing forces. Monologues will not be 'theatre' unless the antagonist, though absent, is implied; unless her *absence* is *present*.

The passion is necessary: theatre, as an art, does not have as its object the commonplace and the trivial, the valueless. It attaches itself to actions in which the characters have an investment, situations in which they venture their lives and their feelings, their moral and their political choices: their passions! What is a passion? It is a feeling for someone or something, or an idea, that we prize more highly than our own life.

And where does the platform fit into all this? In his use of the word 'platform', Lope de Vega reduces all theatres, all existing forms of theatrical architecture, to their simplest equipment and their most elementary expression: a space set apart, a 'place of representation'. This can equally well be a few planks in a public square, an Italian rococo stage, an Elizabethan playhouse or a Spanish 'corral'; today it can be the arena, just as yesterday this was the Greek stage. Modern experiments have transformed lorries, boats, even swimming pools, into theatre stages, and even the stage/audience division has been fragmented in various ways. However, in all cases, separation remains a feature: one space (or more) is intended for the actors and another (or several others) for the spectators, whether these spaces are stationary or mobile.

What is theatre? Boal's expression of Lope de Vega's 'theatre as "two human beings, a passion and a platform"'.

WHAT Is Theatre?
Lope de Vega

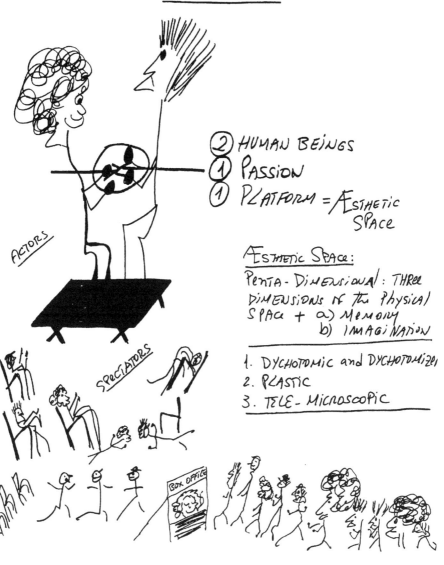

ACTORS

② HUMAN BEINGS
① PASSION
① PLATFORM = ÆSTHETIC SPACE

ÆSTHETIC SPACE:
PENTA-DIMENSIONAL: THREE DIMENSIONS OF THE PHYSICAL SPACE + a) MEMORY
b) IMAGINATION

1. DYCHOTOMIC and DYCHOTOMIZER
2. PLASTIC
3. TELE-MICROSCOPIC

SPECTATORS

BOX OFFICE

Like any space, these various spaces possess, from a physical point of view, three dimensions: length, width and height – the objective dimensions.

Into this empty space, surrounded by things – this stage – other things can enter, other beings. Like the space itself, the things in this space (and the spaces which these things are, every thing being a space) possess these same three physical, objective and measurable dimensions, which are independent of the individuality of each observer. The same surface can seem big to me and small to someone else, but if we measure it we will always find the same square metreage. The same applies to time: an interval of time can seem long to me and short to another; but the number of minutes will be the same.

Spaces possess, then, subjective dimensions: an affective dimension and an oneiric⊚ dimension, which we will study later.

⊚ Oneiric – of or belonging to dreams.

THE AESTHETIC SPACE

The object which Lope de Vega calls the 'platform' has as its primary function the creation of a *separation*, a *division* between the space of the actor – the one who *acts* – and the space of the spectator – the one who *observes* (spectare = to see).

However, this separation becomes more important *per se* than the object which produces it. It can occur even without that object. The separation of spaces can occur without the 'platform' existing as an actual object. All that is required is that, within the bounds of a certain space, spectators and actors designate a more restricted space as 'stage': an aesthetic⊚ space. Whatever the process by which the bounds of this limited space have been determined, we then accept it as an aesthetic space, and it acquires all of the concomitant properties, even in the absence of a physical platform or any other object; it is a space within a space, a superposition of spaces. It can be a corner of the room, or a space around a tree in the open air. We simply decide that 'here' is 'the stage' and the rest of the room, or the rest of whatever space is being used, is 'the auditorium': a smaller space within a larger space. The interpenetration of these two spaces is the *aesthetic space*.

⊚ In its Greek root 'aesthetic' means, 'of or pertaining to things perceptible by the senses'.

An overlaying of spaces; a space is created subjectively by the gaze of the spectators – witnesses present or imagined – inside a space which already existed physically, in three dimensions. The latter is contemporaneous with the spectator; the former travels in time.◉

The aesthetic space thus comes into being because the combined attention of a whole audience converges upon it; it attracts, centripetally, like a black hole. This force of attraction is aided by the very structure of theatres and the positioning of stages, which oblige the spectators all to look in the same direction; and it is abetted by the simple presence of actors and spectators who connive in their acceptance of the theatrical codes and their participation in the celebration of the show. The 'theatre-platform' is a 'time-space'; it exists as such and will retain its particular properties as long as spectators are present or implied.

Thus we can say that not even the physical presence of spectators is necessary for the creation of this subjectively dimensioned space: it will suffice for actors – or a single actor, even a single person – to animate the real or virtual existence of that space and be aware of it. Anyone can designate and thereby create such a space, in their own front room, a space which occupies part or all of the room and immediately becomes, 'aesthetically', a 'stage': the 'platform'. The creator of such a space can then play for herself, without an audience – or with an imaginary audience – like an actor rehearsing alone in an empty theatre: in front of the future audience, absent at that moment, but present in the imagination.

So theatre does not exist in the objectivity of bricks and mortar, sets and costumes, but in the subjectivity of those who practise it, at the moment when they practise it. It needs neither stage nor audience; the actor will suffice. With the actor is born the theatre. The actor is theatre. We are all actors: we are theatre!

Aesthetic space exists whenever there is either separation between the actor's space and the spectator's, or dissociation of two times – 'today I am here and yesterday I was here'. Or today and tomorrow; or now and before; or now and later. We coincide with ourselves when we integrate, into the present we are living, our memory of the past and our imagination of the future. (To coincide with ourselves is to be two in one, as we are on stage.)

The 'theatre' (or 'platform', at its simplest, or 'aesthetic space', at its purest) serves as a means of separating actor from spectator; the one who acts from the one who observes. Actor and spectator can be two different people; they can also *coincide in the same person.*

◉ The great similarity between aesthetic spaces in non-theatre contexts and the aesthetic space of theatre gives rise to the fact that when such spaces occur in reality we speak of 'the theatre of events' (for example, 'Beirut was the theatre of these bloody events; Bosnia was the theatre of war'): we look objectively at the physical space where a catastrophe has taken place and try subjectively to imagine it in all its details.

We have seen that for theatre to exist, neither stage nor spectators are necessary. And we can affirm that even actors – in the professional, full-time sense – are not necessary to it, since aesthetic activity, which emanates from the aesthetic space, is 'vocational', it belongs to all human beings and manifests itself constantly in our relations with other people and other objects. This activity is concentrated a thousand times and made a thousandfold more intense in what we call theatre or performance.

Since the division between stage and audience is not only spatial and architectural, but also intensely subjective, it dampens, discourages, de-activates the 'audience' part and confers on the 'stage' part two subjective dimensions: the affective dimension and the oneiric dimension. The affective dimension is principally responsible for the introduction of memory into the aesthetic space, while the oneiric dimension brings imagination into play.

CHARACTERISTICS AND PROPERTIES OF THE AESTHETIC SPACE

The aesthetic space possesses gnoseological properties, that is, properties which stimulate knowledge and discovery, cognition and recognition: properties which stimulate the process of learning by experience. Theatre is a form of knowledge.

THE FIRST PROPERTY OF THE AESTHETIC SPACE: PLASTICITY

In the aesthetic space one can be without being. Dead people are alive, the past becomes present, the future is today, duration is dissociated from time, everything is possible in the here-and-now, fiction is pure reality, and reality is fiction.

All combinations are possible there, because the aesthetic space *is* but *doesn't exist.* . . .® A battered old chair will be a king's throne, a cross becomes a cathedral, the branch of a tree a forest, and time flows as easily forwards as backwards; the chairs mutate into planes and the cross into a gun; time is not measured; only duration counts, and even location changes. Time and space can be condensed or stretched at will, and the same flexibility operates with people and objects, which can coalesce or dissolve, divide or multiply.

This extreme plasticity allows and encourages total creativity.

® In contrast to physical space which *exists*, but which, in the terms of the aesthetic space, *is not*: the stage *exists* as a stage, but for the duration of the show it is not a stage but the kingdom of Denmark.

The aesthetic space is endowed with the same plasticity as dreams and possesses the same substantiality of physical dimensions and solidity of volumes. We are 'there' in the dream just as the aesthetic space is 'here and now'. That is why, in theatre, we can have concrete dreams.

The aesthetic space liberates memory and imagination

Memory is comprised of all the ideas we have ever had, all the sensations and emotions we have ever experienced, which remain stored within us. 'I remember . . . !' We are in the domain of the real: 'That happened to me! I experienced it! And that's the way it happened!' (Let me draw the reader's attention to the fact that 'I remember this or that' is a solitary act, while 'I recall this or that' is a dialogue.)

Imagination, by contrast, is a process of amalgamation involving all these ideas, emotions and sensations. Here we are in the realms of the possible, if we accept that it is possible to think of impossibilities. Imagination – the sign or premonition of a reality – is, in itself, a reality. Memory and imagination form part of the same psychic process: one does not exist without the other. I could not imagine if I did not have a memory. I cannot recall something without imagination, since memory itself forms part of the process of imagination (I imagine seeing what I have seen, hearing what I have heard, thinking again what I have thought before, etc.). The one is retrospective, the other is prospective.

Memory and imagination project on to – and into – the aesthetic space subjective dimensions which are absent in physical space.

The affective dimension and the oneiric dimension

These two dimensions of space exist only within the mind of the subject. They are projected on to a space in which they are not immanent. The creation of aesthetic space is a human faculty; animals have no access to it. An animal does not 'come on stage'; it is led on to the stage, which it doesn't recognise as such, since it lives always in a single space, the physical.

The affective dimension fills the aesthetic space with new significations and awakens in each observer, in divers forms and intensities, emotions, sensations and thoughts. The return of two adult brothers to the family home of their childhood will not produce in them the same ideas, emotions, sensations and thoughts. The sensations of an estate agent who is valuing this house will be at even greater variance: he will be thinking in terms of dollars, while one brother is thinking of his first kiss and the other of his dead mother. And yet the same house is the trigger for all three meditations.

In the affective dimension, the observer observes, the spectator sees: she feels, is moved, thinks, remembers, imagines. She remains a subject, separate from her object. The affective space thus created is dichotomic, but also asynchronous: it is at one and the same time *what it is* and *what it has been*, or what it could have been, or what it could become. It is in the present, but also in the remembered past or the imagined future. In the present, the observer sees the past – or simulates the future – which she juxtaposes with her current perceptions.

In the oneiric dimension, on the other hand, the observer is drawn of her own volition into the vertigo of the dream, she loses contact with the concrete, real, physical space. Oneiric space is not dichotomic because, in dreaming, we lose our consciousness of the physical space in which we, the dreamers, are dreaming. Though the body may be immobile, we are drawn into the space of the dream, whether we are asleep or awake, whether we have our eyes closed or are at that moment seeing what stimulates our reverie, prompts or triggers our hallucination.

In the affective dimension, the subject observes the physical space and projects onto it his memories and his sensibility. He remembers situations lived or desired, successes and failures; he is swayed by everything he knows, and also by all that dwells obstinately in his unconscious. In the oneiric dimension, the dreamer does not observe: here she penetrates into her own projections, she passes through the looking-glass; everything merges and mixes together, anything is possible.

THE SECOND PROPERTY OF THE AESTHETIC SPACE: IT IS DICHOTOMIC AND IT CREATES DICHOTOMY

This property is born out of the fact that we are dealing with a space within a space: two spaces occupy the same place, at the same time. The people and the things which are in this place will be in two spaces.[◉]

These spaces are identical and different. Identical because we are breathing the same air in the auditorium and on the stage, and the same lighting is illuminating both actor and character. Identical because, artists and spectators alike, we are concretely in the same time in the same town. Different because on stage the illusion of an unfamiliar and distant world is created, while in the auditorium, here and now, we accept and live this illusion. Different because on stage one acts and in the auditorium one observes.

The aesthetic space is dichotomic and creates dichotomy, and all those who penetrate it become dichotomic there. On stage the actor is who he is and who he seems to be. He is here and now, in front of us, but he is also far away from us, in another place, in another time, where the story he is telling and experiencing is taking place; he is Sergio Cardoso,[◉] or John Gielgud, and he is Hamlet. Being a space which creates dichotomy, the aesthetic space dichotomises the spectators: we are here, seated in this very room, and at the same time we are in the castle of Elsinore.

◉ By way of empirical proof of this, we can cite the common experience of being in the audience at a theatre when our neighbours are talking out loud and we momentarily abandon Hamlet's Denmark to shut them up: we are in the auditorium and in the kingdom. Two bodies cannot simultaneously occupy the same place in space. On the other hand, a single body can be in two spaces at the same time; all that is required is an aesthetic space within the physical space.

◉ Sergio Cardoso was one of Brazil's leading classical actors in the 1950s.

The theatrical stage and the therapeutic stage

In a 'Stanislavskian' production, the actor knows she is an actor, but consciously tries to be unaware of the presence of the audience. In a Brechtian production, the actor is completely aware of the presence of the audience, which she transforms into genuine interlocutors, but mute interlocutors. (So even in this case, soliloquy is the form we are dealing with. Only in a Forum Theatre show do the spectators acquire voice and movement, sound and colour, and thus become able to demonstrate their ideas and desires. That is why the Theatre of the Oppressed was invented.)

Whatever the form of theatre, the actor always establishes a binary relationship with the character she is playing – attraction and repulsion, fusion and dissociation. According to style or theatrical genre, the distance between actor and character can increase or diminish. In drama or tragedy, this distance diminishes; in comedy or farce it increases. It diminishes in a Stanislavskian performance and increases in a Brechtian performance. It is smaller for the actor, greater for the clown.

Whether greater or smaller, this distance always exists. On stage, an actor, though entirely immersed in his deepest emotions, is completely aware of his actions. However moved he may be, he always maintains a total control over himself. Playing Othello, only a madman – never an actor! – could actually strangle the actress playing Desdemona. The actor does not deprive himself of the pleasure of killing the character, but he preserves the physical integrity of the actress.

This is what happens on a theatre stage and, in a similar fashion, on a therapeutic stage. Here too the dichotomic and 'dichotomising' properties of the aesthetic space take root and exercise their powers.

In the first case, the protagonist-actor produces thoughts and releases emotions and sentiments which, whether her own or not, are supposed to belong to the character, that is to say, someone else. (Later we will study the triad of person–personality–*personnage*.) In the second case, the protagonist-patient (the patient-actor) reproduces her thoughts and releases anew her own emotions and her own sentiments (which are recognised and declared as being her own).

When the protagonist-patient lives a scene in her own life, she tries *to concretise her declared desires*, be they love or hate, attack or flight, construction or destruction. But when she relives the same scene in an aesthetic space (whether theatrical or therapeutic), her desire becomes dichotomic: she wants simultaneously to *show* the scene and to *show herself* in the scene. In showing how the scene was experienced, she is seeking to achieve for a second time the *concretisation*◎ of her desires, as they were realised or frustrated at that time. In showing herself in the scene, she is seeking to make progress towards the actual *concretion*◎ of this desire. *To desire* becomes a *thing*. The verb becomes a palpable noun.

In living the scene, she is trying to concretise a desire; in reliving it, she is reifying it. Her desire, because it is aesthetic, transforms itself into an object which is observable, by herself and by others. The desire, having become a thing, can better be studied, analysed, and (who knows?) transformed. In daily life, the protagonist-actor tries to concretise a declared, conscious desire; the desire to love, for example. In the aesthetic space, she makes the concretion of this love. In this process of reviviscence, not only avowed, overt desires but also unconscious, covert desires become reified. Not only what one wants to reify is reified, but sometimes also things that are there, but hidden.

◎ Concretisation is the putting of the ideas or thoughts into a concrete form, concretion being the actual materialisation of these desires (A.J.).

First time round, a person in her real life, or an actor in rehearsal searching for her character, lives a scene with emotion. Second time round, on the therapeutic or theatrical plane, in front of fellow members of a group or unknown members of an audience, the actor relives the scene with 're-emotion'. The first action is a solitary discovery; the second a revelation, a dialogue.

In both cases, actor and patient are trying to show the 'character' as a 'she', even if, as in the case of the patient, this 'she' is an 'I-before'. In the case of the patient, due to the effect of dichotomy produced by the aesthetic space, we are dealing with two 'I's: the 'I' who is living the scene and the 'I' who is recounting it. This mechanism of reliving allows the simultaneity of an 'I' and an 'other-I', who are separated in space and time and cannot be one – though they are.

This dichotomy obliges the protagonist-patient, since it is herself she is talking about, to choose who she is : ◉is she the 'I' she has been and to whom she is referring (the referent), or is she the present, referring 'I', (the referree), 'I-before' or 'I-now'? The alternative is, however, only apparent; the choice has already been made: the protagonist is the 'I' who tells of the 'I' she has been, since the narrator is a more ample container than the narrated. She could not be the 'I' who lived the scene being recounted (relived), since that would be denying the space and time separating the two scenes: the one which has been lived and the one which is recounted.

This movement forward in space and time is, in itself, therapeutic, since all therapy, before proposing the exercise of a choice, must consist of an inventory of possible alternatives. A process is therapeutic when it allows – and encourages – the patient to choose from several alternatives to the situation in which he finds himself, the situation which causes him unwanted suffering or unhappiness. In enabling, and indeed requiring, the patient to observe himself in action – since his own desire to show obliges him both to *see* and to *see himself* – this theatrical process of recounting, in the present, and in front of witnesses 'in solidarity', a story lived in the past, offers, in itself, an alternative.

In theatric psychotherapies what is important is not the simple entry on stage of the human body, but the effects of the dichotomy which the aesthetic space brings to bear on that body and on the consciousness of the protagonist, who becomes, on stage, subject and object, conscious of himself and his action. In daily life, our

◉ Convention craves that, in the case of the protagonist-actor, the actor be the 'I-now', and the 'I-before' be only a character, a fiction. But we know very well that fiction does not exist, that everything is true. This applies to an even greater extent in the theatre, where even lies are true. The only fiction is the word 'fiction'. And perhaps even the word 'fiction' is true, since it reveals, by antiphrasis, the desire to dissimulate a part of the truth, in declaring it fictitious.

⊚ Similarly, in a Forum Theatre show, members of the audience who come on stage to take the place of the protagonist immediately become the protagonist and thus acquire this dichotomic property: they demonstrate their alternative actions and suggestions, and at the same time, observe the effects and consequences of these alternatives: they evaluate them, reflect on them and think about new tactics and strategies.

This is why, after a Forum Theatre session centred on the individual, the protagonist must not be dispatched back into the auditorium for his actions to be judged or interpreted there – on the contrary, he must be helped to see the people who are seeing him, to observe those who are observing him, to admire (to wonder at) himself with those who are admiring (wondering at) him.

⊚ When I speak of myself, I am the person who is speaking, not the person of whom I speak.

⊚ Ascesis – ἀσκησις – exercise, training. In the Theatre of the Oppressed, ascesis means moving from the phenomenon to the law that regulates all phenomena of the same kind, so as to explain other phenomena that may occur. For instance, an act of aggression against a particular black person is a phenomenon – something which happens only once in a given period of time, even if it is frequently repeated – so, by ascesis, we seek to understand racism, which is the law that explains these phenomena; we try to understand the purposes it serves, and relate this back to all other forms of intolerance. To give an

attention is always – or almost always – directed towards other people or other things. On the 'platform', we direct our attention onto ourselves *as well*. The protagonist acts and observes himself in action, shows and observes himself showing, speaks and listens to what he himself is saying.⊚

In this sense, the invention of theatre is a revolution of Copernican proportions. In our daily lives we are the centre of our universe and we look at facts and people from a single perspective, our own. On stage, we continue to see the world as we have always seen it, but now we also see it as others see it: we see ourselves as we see ourselves, *and* we see ourselves as we are seen. To our own point of view we add others, as if we were able to look at the earth from the earth, where we live, and also from the moon, the sun, a satellite or the stars. In daily life, we see the situation; on stage, we see ourselves and we see the situation we are in.

This dichotomy also allows the protagonist to join forces with the therapist and, possibly, with other members of the group, who together will be able to observe the 'I-before' still present to an extent in 'I-now' – which is, after a fashion, an 'I-again'. But the very process which enables the I-before to be observed, distances it. I see myself yesterday. I am today, yesterday is someone else, an other.⊚ It is one part of me which detaches itself from me in order that I may see it. This part is an object of analysis, of study, aesthetically reified. The protagonist who, in the lived scene, was a subject-*in-situ*, here becomes the subject who is observing a situation in which he is the actual subject: himself yesterday. The 'I-today' can see the 'I-yesterday', the converse obviously not being possible. So, I am now more than I was. In this ascesis,⊚ the protagonist becomes subject of himself and subject of the situation. Within the theatrical fiction, of course. But let us not forget that in the theatre everything is true, even lies. At least, that is our hypothesis.

With the other participants of the group, there occurs a kind of inverse phenomenon. Though they are outside observers, observing from a distance, by virtue of the *sym*-pathy created with the protagonist they become empowered to penetrate into his lived experience and they travel within this protagonist, feeling his emotions and perceiving analogies between their own lives and his, when they exist – and they almost always do exist (only then will there be genuine *sym*-pathy and not mere *em*-pathy). And so they will recognise the points of view of the protagonist and his perspectives.

This phenomenon does not appear in the conventional theatre, since the intransitive relation which holds sway there does not allow the protagonist to respond to a spectator who challenges him. In such a circumstance, the spectator feels as if he is in front of phantoms to which he must surrender empathetically, since they are incapable of reacting to his interpellations. The only transmission is one-way, from stage to auditorium (empathy), without the reciprocal possibility of communion, of dialogue (sympathy).

The importance of theatric therapies does not reside solely in our potential ability to see the individual in action, here and now, in act and word – which is the vision of the therapist. It resides esssentially in this mechanism of transformation of the protagonist, who moves from being the object-subject of social but also psychological forces, conscious and unconscious forces, to become the subject of this object-subject – which is the work of the patient. In this theatric therapy, the patient does the work, assisted of course by the multiple mirror of the observant gaze of all the participants.

THE THIRD PROPERTY OF THE AESTHETIC SPACE: IT IS TELEMICROSCOPIC

On a stage, we see the far-away close up; we see the small made large. The stage brings to today, to here and now, what has happened long ago, far from here: that which had been lost in the mists of time, had deserted memory or fled into unconscious. Like a powerful telescope, the stage brings things closer.

In creating the stage–auditorium division, we transform the stage into a place where everything acquires new dimensions, becomes magnified, as under a powerful microscope. All gestures, all words spoken there, become larger, clearer, more emphatic. On stage it is difficult, almost impossible, to hide.

Thus, brought closer and made larger, human actions can be better observed.

example from the realm of physics: all objects fall to the ground (a phenomenon) so, by ascesis, we understand the law of gravity.

This process of ascesis is one of the tasks of the Joker in a Forum Theatre session and our own task throughout our lives.

CONCLUSION

The extraordinary gnoseological (knowledge-enhancing) power of theatre is due to these three essential properties: (1) plasticity, which allows and induces the unfettered exercise of memory and imagination, the free play of past and future; (2) the division or doubling of self which occurs in the subject who comes on stage, the fruit of the dichotomic and 'dichotomising' character of the 'platform', which allows – and enables – self-observation; (3) finally, that telemicroscopic property which magnifies everything and makes everything present, allowing us to see things which, without it, in smaller or more distant form, would escape our gaze.

These properties are aesthetic, that is to say, related to the senses. Knowledge is acquired here via the senses and not solely via the mind. Before all else, we see and we listen, and it is thanks to this that we understand (sight and hearing being the principal senses mediating in theatrical communication). The specific therapeutic function of the theatre resides in this: seeing and hearing. In seeing and listening – and in seeing oneself and listening to oneself – the protagonist acquires knowledge about himself. I see and I see myself, I speak and I listen to myself, I think and I think about myself; all of which is only possible because of the doubling of the 'I': I-now' perceives 'I-before' and has a presentiment of (anticipates) a 'possible-I', a 'future-I'.

This doubling, certainly possible in other spaces, is here, on stage, inevitable, intense: aesthetic. This process of knowledge, this specific, artistic therapy, is constituted not only of ideas but also of emotions and sensations. Theatre is a therapy into which one enters body and soul, soma and psyche.

It is interesting to note that the word 'psyche', which designates the whole ensemble of psychic phenomena that go to make up a personal unity, also designates a 'cheval glass', a fixed-base, mobile mirror the angle of which can be adjusted to allow one to see one's whole body.

In the psyche/mirror one sees one's body; in one's body (in the theatre) one sees one's psyche.

In the psyche/mirror one sees one's psyche; one sees oneself in the other.

Theatre is this psyche/mirror where we can see our psyche.

Theatre holds 'a mirror up to nature' (Shakespeare). And the

Theatre of the Oppressed is a mirror which we can penetrate to modify our image!

What is the human being?

The most important of the three elements in Lope de Vega's definition of theatre is, of course, the human being. It is impossible to imagine a play, or even a scene, without the presence of a human being.

For example, let us imagine a show which begins with some marvellous lighting effects, controlled by a state-of-the-art computer, lights which blaze on and off creating a harmony of colour and sensation, all this orchestrated with divine music, a 'stereo-sensurround' sound system. In the middle of the stage, a superb table, draped in black lace, and in the middle of the table a black pistol. Thus begins the play and so it goes on for one, two, three, five minutes. Sounds and colours, colours and lights, lights and sound, for ten, twenty minutes. And so on. However beautiful the music, however stupendous the colours and the kaleidoscopic lights, however perfect the lines of table, tablecloth and pistol, of all the props and all the décor, how long will the public stay in the auditorium?

It lacks something. It lacks the human being, whose absence is permissible only for a short period of time.

However, it only needs someone – man or woman – to make an appearance and theatre will inhabit the stage. If he or she approaches the table, the theatricality is intensified. If he or she lays hands on the pistol, the theatrical temperature will rise, and it will continue to rise if he/she points the pistol at his/her head. It will rise even higher, considerably higher, if he/she points it at the audience! By this point we will have intense theatre. So, from this we can conclude that theatre is essentially the human being.

But what is the human being? The human being, first and foremost, is a body. Whatever our religious inclination, I am sure that we would all accept that there is no human being without a human body. And this body – this human body that we are – has five main properties:

1. it is sensitive
2. it is emotive
3. it is rational

4. it has a sex

5. it can move

Unlike stones and metals, unlike 'things', living creatures experience sensations. This sensitivity reaches its pinnacle in the human being. The human body registers sensations and consequently reacts. These sensations are possible thanks to our five senses.

The senses have connections with each other. Moreover, our sensations are registered in our brain. If I am walking along and stumble on a stone, the sensation I feel does not leave my mind – I experienced the sensation in my foot but my head registers it. Everything I feel (what I feel in my skin, what I hear, what I see, the odours I smell or the tastes I taste) I feel in my five senses and I feel with my brain. (If further proof is needed, here is one, unhappily both definitive and unverifiable! If someone chopped off our head, we would no longer sense anything, neither perfumes of Arabia nor kicks on the shins.)

Were we scientists, we would now be obliged to undertake a more in-depth study of the brain, the nervous system and each of its constituent elements; we would have to apply ourselves to a study of the manner in which sensations experienced by the body are registered in the brain. But, as artists practising theatre, it will suffice for us to state that this process takes place, in some region or other of our brain. Our whole body ends up there, coordinates itself there, is logged there.

The body is also emotive, and sensations of pleasure or pain can lead us to emotions of love, hate or fear, or any other emotion. In the human being, all sensation arouses emotion. Equally, the human being is a rational creature, it knows things, it is capable of thinking, of understanding, and of making mistakes. These three 'regions' – the sites of our sensations, our emotions and our thoughts – are not like countries marked on a map, each with its own colour and its own frontiers: communication between them is free and exchange continuous; sensations transform themselves into emotions and these then give rise to specific thoughts. But this traffic is genuinely reversible, the channels are two-way; thoughts provoke emotions and emotions sensations.

To illustrate the first case, we can cite the example of a baby who is hungry and because of his hunger (a sensation), cries with irritation (an emotion) but smiles when he sees his mother enter the room because he understands that he is going to be fed (reason). Mum was not there, now she is: this is reason, an act of cognition, these are ideas. He was irritated, on edge, he was afraid, now he is smiling, happy; these are emotions. And even if he still has an empty stomach and feels pain because he is hungry, the emotion of happiness caused by the simple presence of the maternal breast already makes him experience more pleasant sensations.

For the path which leads from reason to sensation, we can use Einstein by way of example. One day, he experienced the illumination of a dazzling discovery: $E = MC^2$. As abstract an idea as could be imagined, almost unthinkable for most mere mortals, this formula establishes a relationship between mass and energy, with the mediation of the square of the speed of light. The story goes that when Einstein thought up this combination of letters and figures he was immediately prey to torrential and contradictory emotions. He experienced happiness because of his discovery and pity towards the scientist whose theories he had just destroyed. 'Newton, forgive me!' he stammered through trembling lips, in a presentiment of atomic slaughter and at the same time rejoicing in anticipation of his future discoveries. A tumult of emotions and sensations, produced simply by this very abstract idea: $E = MC^2$.

So we arrive at a division of the brain into three regions, without concerning ourselves too much with anatomical or physiological accuracy: the region of sensations, the region of emotions, and the region of thoughts. Suppose we imagine that these regions are located side by side, separated by vertical lines. We would be entitled to ask ourselves whether the upper part of our schema is identical to the lower part. It is not! We must once again divide the brain into three regions, but this time with the lines drawn horizontally. On top, the conscious mind, the verbalised; in the middle, the verbalisable; right at the bottom, the unconscious.

In fact, we are conscious of a great number of sensations, emotions and ideas. We know that it is either cold or hot; we know that we hate injustice; we are conscious of what we think needs to be done to enable so many oppressed people to liberate themselves from so much oppression. Sometimes this is very clear in our minds, and we are conscious of it. But what does 'to be conscious of something' mean? It means that we are capable of explaining, of putting into words. We can say we are conscious of something when we are capable of explaining it – however well or

WHAT IS A HUMAN BEING?

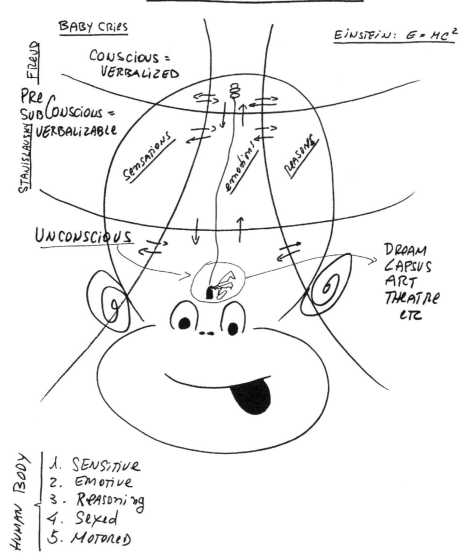

BABY CRIES

CONSCIOUS =
VERBALIZED

EINSTEIN: $E = MC^2$

FREUD

STANISLAVSKY

PRE
SUBCONSCIOUS =
VERBALIZABLE

Sensations

emotions

Reasons

UNCONSCIOUS

DREAM
LAPSUS
ART
THEATRE
ETC

HUMAN BODY
1. SENSITIVE
2. EMOTIVE
3. REASONING
4. SEXED
5. MOTORED

↑ What is a human being?

What is an actor? Here Boal shows the pressure cooker of the person, stimulated by the fire of theatre, the nozzles/outlets being controlled by fear and moral(ity). We see the angels that emerge – the personality, the controlled face we show to the world – and the devils – the dramatis personae, the characters that theatre can coax out.

badly – totally or in part. We may explain it better or worse, just as we are more or less conscious of it.

Below this first horizontal region we can place a second region, to which Stanislavski gave the name 'sub-conscious' and which Freud called, in his early works, the 'pre-conscious'. This region is the dwelling place of ideas, emotions and sensations which are capable of verbalisation but are not actually verbalised. They do not quite find their way into conscious memory, but neither have they fallen completely into oblivion. They are forgotten, or hidden, but they can re-emerge into the light.

Finally, at the base of these zones, the most secret region: the unconscious, that which is not verbalised and which, in its depths, will never be capable of verbalisation. The hidden part, in unfathomable waters, never to be revealed.

As with the vertical divisions, this hypothesis of horizontal lines does not establish precise frontiers; the possibility of circulation exists. (We seek above all to engineer circulation from the bottom to the top, to bring to light the subterranean or sunken treasures resting in these murky depths.)

In the absence of precise, hermetic, compartmentalised borders, that which was conscious can become pre- or un-conscious; and that which was unconscious can rise back up to the surface and become word. These are slender, fragile layers, one on top of another, darker towards the bottom, clearer towards the top. These sensations, emotions and ideas, whether exposed to the light of day or fled into the shadows, are always alive, always active, and all the more terrible the darker they are, all the more uncontrollable for dwelling in darkness.

The depths of the unconscious are difficult to access: we do not reach them by speech alone. But we can get there by means of the dream, that *royal road to the unconscious*, as Freud called it, by means of hallucinations, word-games, slips of the tongue and act, and also by myths, by the arts, by the theatre. The great works of theatre penetrate directly into our unconscious and enter into dialogue with it. It is not out of interest in Pericles' Greece that we are fascinated by *Oedipus Rex*, it is out of interest in ourselves: Oedipus speaks of us, speaks for us, speaks in us.

So much for the human being. Some human beings are actors. To explain the human being is a Herculean, gigantic task; to explain the actor is almost impossible.

Let's try!

What is the actor?

The human being is – to a limited extent and with a large margin of error – a knowable entity; we know more about its body than its psyche. We know a certain amount about some elements of the workings of its psyche, those that relate to consciousness. And we have some hypotheses, some conjectures about those that do not.

We can compare the unconscious to a pressure-cooker. All manner of demons bubble away inside it: all the saints, all the vices, all the virtues, everything that, not being act, exists in potential. Each of us has, within him, everything that all other men, all other women have; Eros and Thanatos. We have loyalty and treachery, courage and cowardice, bravery and fear. We desire life and death, for ourselves and for others. We have the whole gamut, in pure potentiality, boiling away, in a hermetically sealed pan. We have within us such a wealth of possibilities! And we know so very little of it, so little about what we have, and almost nothing about what we are!

All possibilities being within us, it is impossible for us to manifest this potential in its totality. Within us, we have every-thing, we are a *person*. But this *person* is so rich and so powerful, so intense, with such a multiplicity of forms and faces, that we are constrained to reduce it. This suppression of our freedom of expression and action results from two causes: external, social coercion and/or internal, ethical choice. Fear and morality. I do or do not do thousands of things, I behave or do not behave in thousands of different ways because I am constrained by social factors, which force me to be this or stop me from being that.

This assortment of factors includes police and family, univer-sities and churches, judges and advertisers. They tell us what is permitted and what is forbidden. And, for the most part, we accept it. Or equally, we define ourselves and oblige ourselves to be what we are, to do what we do, not to do what we think is wrong. There is one external morality, conditioned by the outside world, and another internal morality conditioned by habit. Both forces, a welter of obligations and interdictions, constrain us. We always remain the *person* we are, but we only transform a tiny portion of our potentiality into *acts*. I shall call this reduction *personality*.

We all have a *personality*, which is a reduction forced out of our *person*. The latter boils on in the saucepan; the former escapes through the safety valve. And, in this fashion, we scrape along perfectly well. Because we pretend to be only that part of ourselves which is excusable; the rest we keep carefully hidden. However, both our demons and our saints remain alive, very much alive, at boiling point, and they may declare their presence by means of symptoms, ulcers, rashes or other, even worse, manifestations. Nevertheless, to all appearances we are healthy smiling people.

Now let us take an actor, the very incarnation of smiling sanity. Suppose all her material problems are solved, she has long contracts, large salaries; she has simple and normal preoccupations. Suppose, then, that we are talking about someone 'normal', that is, according to the socially accepted norms defining 'normal' people.

This normal actor pursues a strange and perilous occupation: she interprets parts in plays, characters, dramatis personae. Where can she go to find them?

And, before we go any further, who are they, these people we call 'characters'? Let's be frank: from a medical point of view, they are all neurotics, psychotics, paranoiacs, melancholics, schizophrenics: in short, sick people! As literature, sure, they are enthralling; but in reality, they would be in urgent need of medical attention. Characters in plays are sick people: this generalisation we can make without fear of error. And it is for this single reason that we go to the theatre. I have seen *Hamlet* dozens of times, I love the play and its eponymous protagonist, but I am not sure if I would want to invite him round to dinner every Saturday, along with other friends, to spend the evening chatting about being or not being.

Take the following scenario. Who would want to go out to go and see a piece of theatre like this? A young man and a young woman, both good-looking and in good health, in love with each other, watch their children getting ready for school, where they are by far the best pupils. They accompany them to the school gate. Then they cross a flower-filled garden under the admiring and sympathetic gaze of their friendly neighbours, when, all of a sudden – here comes the postman! Hold onto your hats . . . he is the bearer of glad tidings – both mothers-in-law are in perfect health, and they are on a cruise around the Greek islands, and the weather is good. . . .

Who would happily sit through such a play? No one! Not even Doris Day would perform in such a play. The only audience in such a theatre would be flies. The thing that prompts us to go to the theatre is conflict, combat; we want to see mad people and fanatics, thieves and murderers. And, I accept, a smattering of good souls, just enough to set off the evil in all its glory. We hunger for the strange, the abnormal.

And so our actor – of sound mind – must play a sick character. Where then can she go to seek such a character? Not into her personality, which is, as we know, exempt from evil, but into her person, deep within, right inside, in the pressure-cooker, the place where the demons dwell at boiling point. And the actor, having patiently tamed her wildcats long ago, is once again obliged to go and waken them. That is why the profession of actor is so unhealthy and so dangerous. I swear, actors should be entitled to the same danger money allowances as miners seeking out coal or tin in the depth of mines, or astronauts who have to fly to vertiginous and infinite heights. Actors search the depths of the soul and the infinity of the metaphysical.◎ Bless them!

Actors taunt the lion with a blade of grass.◎ Their *personalities*, a picture of health and sanity, go looking in their *persons* for sick people and demons – the dramatis personae or *personnages* (French) – in the hope that, once the curtain has fallen, they will be able to get them back into their cages. And, in the best of hypotheses, they succeed in doing this. They always try, and when they succeed, they enjoy a catharsis. But sometimes – and it is tragic when it happens! – once awoken, Iago and Tartuffe, having discovered the bright limelights, also want to know the light of day, and refuse to return to the darkness of that Pandora's box which each of us is. There are actors who become ill. Our profession is truly unhealthy!

But whether dangerous or not, it is there, in the depths of the person, that the actor is obliged to seek out her characters. Otherwise, she would be a mere conjurer or jongleur, playing with her characters, but with no proximity to them; a puppet-master controlling her puppets, at a safe distance. Or, at its most extreme, a manipulator of mannequins, whose contact with her characters is hardly skin-deep. No. The actor does not work with mannequins, marionettes, balls or rods. The actor works with human beings, and therefore works with herself, on the infinite process of discovering the human. In this way alone can she justify her art. The other would be the sort of craftsmanship which, though perfectly commendable, is not art. Craftsmanship reproduces pre-existing models; art discovers essences.

Sarah Bernhardt, speaking of her creative process, wrote:

◎ Theatre is the fire which makes the pressure-cooker explode and release the angels and devils dwelling inside it.

◎ Brazilian expression meaning 'to tempt fate'.

> Little by little, I used to identify with my character. I used to dress her with great care and leave my Sarah Bernhardt in a corner of the dressing room: I made her into a spectator of my new 'self'; and I went on stage ready to suffer, cry, laugh, love, unaware of what the 'I' of my 'other self' was doing up in my dressing room.

Sarah Bernhardt, *The Art of Theatre*, p.204.

To sum up, the healthy personality of the actor searches out, in the richness of her person, her characters or *personnages*, beings less healthy than herself, sick people.

Thus, within the limits of the scene and the moment, the free exercise of all asocial tendencies, unacceptable desires, forbidden behaviours and unhealthy feelings is allowed. On stage, all is permissible, nothing is forbidden. The demons and saints which inhabit the person of the actor are completely free to blossom, to experience the orgasm of the show, to pass from potential into act. In a mimetic and emphatic fashion, the same thing happens with the analogous demons and saints which are awakened in the hearts of the spectators. Always in the hope that, after it is all over, they will be tired out and will go back to sleep. In the hope that, in this holy and diabolic ball, the saints and demons of actors and audience will return, exhausted, to the unconscious darkness of the person, restoring the health and equilibrium of the personalities, which will then be able, without fear, to reintegrate their lives into society. In the hope that after the carnivalesque paroxysms of theatre will come once again the Ash Wednesday of a new day's work.

These new techniques, such as The Cop in the Head and Rainbow of Desire, as with the Theatre of the Oppressed as a whole, advance the hypothesis that the same path can be travelled, in an inverse manner, with different, even opposite, objectives.

To be an actor is dangerous, yes, but why? Because the catharsis that one seeks is not inevitable. For all the security his profession gives him, for all the protection offered by the rituals of theatre, for all the established theories about what is fiction and what is reality, none of this can prevent the possibility that one day these aroused personalities (characters, *personnages*) may refuse to go quietly back to sleep, these lions may refuse to return to their cages in the zoo of our souls.

If that is the case, we can envisage the contrary hypothesis: a sick personality can, in theory, try to awaken healthy *personnages*, this time not with the goal of dispatching them back into oblivion but in the hope of mixing them into his personality. I am afraid, but inside me there also lives the courageous man; if I can wake him up, perhaps I could keep him awake.

Who is the 'I'? The person, the personality or the *personnage*? It is very easy for us to decide – in fatalistic fashion – that we are the way we are, full stop, end of story. But we can also imagine – in a more creative fashion – that the playing cards can be re-dealt.

In this dance of potentialities, different powers take the floor at different times – potential can become act, occupy the spotlight and then glide back to the sidelines, powers grow and diminish, move in to the foreground and then shrink into the background again – everything is mutable. Our personality is what it is, but it is also what it is becoming. If we are fatalists, then there is nothing to be done; but if we are not, we can try.

In this book I give some examples of this. Without dogmatism. Without triumphalism. Without wishful thinking. To tell the truth, without being absolutely sure. But with enormous hope. A well-founded hope: if the actor can become a sick person, the sick person can in turn become a healthy actor.

3 THE THREE HYPOTHESES OF 'THE COP IN THE HEAD'

In a Theatre of the Oppressed session, there are no *spectators*, only *active observers* (or spect-actors). The centre of gravity is in the auditorium, not on the stage. An image or scene which does not reverberate for the observers cannot be worked on with these techniques, because it will be about a wholly personal, non-pluralisable, case.

The Theatre of the Oppressed has two fundamental linked principles: it aims (a) to help the spect-actor transform himself into a protagonist of the dramatic action and rehearse alternatives for his situation, so that he may then be able (b) to extrapolate into his real life the actions he has rehearsed in the practice of theatre.

In order to bring about these primary objectives, the Theatre of the Oppressed as a whole and the Cop in the Head system in particular suggest three fundamental hypotheses.

First hypothesis: osmosis

The smallest cells of social organisation (the couple, the family, the neighbourhood, the school, the office, the factory, etc.) and equally the smallest incidents of our social life (an accident at the corner of the street, the checking of identity papers in the metro, a visit to the doctor, etc.) contain all the moral and political values of society, all its structures of domination and power, all its mechanisms of oppression.

The great general themes are inscribed in the small personal themes and incidents. When we talk about a strictly individual case, we are also talking about the generality of similar cases and we are talking about the society in which this particular case can occur.

All the singular elements of the individual story must acquire a *symbolic* character, and shed the constraints of singularity, unique-ness. Thus by generalisation, and not by singularisation, we abandon a terrain which is more apt for study by psychothera-pists and limit ourselves to that which is our terrain and our privilege: the art of theatre.

Twenty years ago, an interesting experiment was carried out in the United States, in the segregationist South and in New York where integration was further advanced. White, green, blue and black dolls were shown to black children. They were asked to choose from these the prettiest and the ugliest. In the South, where the 'segregated' blacks kept a firmer grip on their own values, the children said that the prettiest was the black one and the ugliest the white one. In the North, where integration imposes the values of white society, the outcome was the reverse: the white one was the pretty one and the black one the ugly one. The black children had acquired white values.

This propagation of ideas, of values, of tastes, I will call *osmosis*: interpenetration.

How does osmosis come about? As much by repression as by seduction. Through repulsion, hatred, fear, violence, constraint, or, by contrast, through attraction, love, desire, promises, dependences, etc.

Where does osmosis emerge? Everywhere. In all the cells of our social life. In the family (through parental legal power, money, dependence, affectivity), in work (through wages, bonuses, holidays, unemployment, retirement, etc.), in the army (punishment, promotion, rank, the seduction of the exercise of power, etc.), in school (marks, end-of-year rankings, reports . . .), advertising (through the false association of ideas: beautiful women and cigarettes, the Niagara Falls and whisky), in the newspapers (the selection of news items, the manipulation of diagrams), in the Church (Hell, Paradise, fate, communion, forgiveness, sin, hope).

Also in the theatre. How?

The mainstream theatre juxtaposes two worlds: the world of the audience and that of the stage. The conventional rituals of the theatre determine the roles to be played by the former and the latter. On stage images of social life are presented in an organic, autonomous fashion, in such a way that the audience may not alter them. During the show, the audience is de-activated, reduced to contemplation (even if this contemplation is sometimes critical) of the events unfolding on the stage.

Osmosis takes place, in an intransitive way, from stage to audience. If there is a very strong resistance in the audience to letting itself be de-activated, the show can come to a halt, but it cannot change, because it is predetermined.

The conventional theatrical ritual is conservative, *immobiliste*, opposed to progress. Certainly, through this conservatism, this *immobilisme*, a play can *transmit* − the movement still being intransitive – ideas which are *mobilising*. But the ritual itself remains immobilising.

Cervantes' play, *Numance*, tells the story of a town under siege whose inhabitants have decided to resist to the very last man, woman and child. They are massacred, but they do not surrender. During the Spanish civil war, *Numance* was performed in a town under siege from the Fascists. Evidently the show produced a fantastic mobilising effect, even if the theatrical ritual itself remained immobilising. In this particular case, reality violently shattered the ritual. In a normal show we usually forget about external reality; we have to concentrate our attention on the stage. Here the stage only reminded the audience of what was going on in the street. The *immobilisme* of the theatrical ritual was broken by the dynamism of the events of the social world.

In the Theatre of the Oppressed, we try to invert this *immobilisme*, to *make the dialogue between stage and audience totally transitive*, in both directions: the stage can try to transform the audience, but the audience can also transform everything, try anything.

This transmission is not always pacific. It is founded on the subject–object relationship. But noone can be reduced to the condition of absolute object. So, the oppressor produces in the oppressed two types of reaction: submission and subversion. *Every oppressed person is a subjugated subversive*. His submission is his Cop in the Head, his introjection. But he also possesses the other element, subversion. Our goal is to dynamise the latter, by making the former disappear.

Second hypothesis: metaxis

In a traditional theatre show, the *spectator–character* (or spectator–actor) relationship comes into being by means of what is called *empathy. em*, inside, *pathos*, emotion.

The emotion of the characters penetrates us, the moral world of the show invades us, osmotically; we are led by characters and actions not under our control; we experience a *vicarious* emotion.

In a Theatre of the Oppressed showing, where the oppressed themselves have created their own world of images of their own oppressions, the *active observer (spect-actor)–character* relationship changes in essence and becomes *sympathy: sym*, with. We are not led, we lead. I am not penetrated by the emotion of others; instead

I project my own. I guide my own actions, I am the subject. Or else someone like me guides the action: we are both subjects.

In the first case, the shifting stage sweeps me along with it; in the second, it is I that shift it.

The oppressed becomes the artist.

The oppressed-artist produces a world of art. She creates images of her real life, of her real oppressions. This world of images contains, *aesthetically transubstantiated*, the same oppressions that exist in the real world that prompted these images.

When the oppressed herself, in the role of artist, creates images of her own oppressive reality, she belongs to both these worlds utterly and completely, not merely 'vicariously'. Here we see the phenomenon of *metaxis*: the state of belonging completely and simultaneously to two different, autonomous worlds: the image of reality and the reality of the image. She shares and belongs to these two autonomous worlds: her reality and the image of her reality, which she herself has created.

It is vital that these two worlds be truly autonomous. The artistic creativity of the oppressed-protagonist must not limit itself to simple realistic reproduction or symbolic illustration of the actual oppression: *it must have its own aesthetic dimension.*

Frequently, the participants insist on the *signification* of each image. This means that they are calling for the *translation* of an image (which belongs to a particular language, the language of images) into another language, the language of idiom, verbal language. But it should be noted that images do not translate – no more than the opening chords of Beethoven's Fifth can be translated as *destiny knocks at the door*, as someone has already attempted to do, in a 500-page book.

There are many people who have difficulty in enjoying abstract painting because they always try to interpret, to translate the images. If a painting is called 'Still life', these people try to make out the grapes, to locate the pineapples, or the bananas . . . as in Picasso's picture 'Femme nue avec pomme', when one tries to spot the woman, or at least the apple, and one finds neither one nor the other. The woman and the apple no longer exist in their original substance: in the picture they are transubstantiated. Now they exist only in Picasso's head. Metaxis occurs in him, inside him. By means of *sym*-pathy, we have to identify with Picasso himself, and then metaxis will occur in us too: we will be able to paint a similar picture. Or at least, enjoy Picasso's picture. . . .

If our society, our culture, our social life have nothing to do with Picasso's, metaxis will not occur in us, because our transitive identification (our sympathy) with him will be impossible. It would be difficult for someone from China or Chile to have the same experience in front of this picture, to enjoy the same species of pleasure, as a French person or a European of the same social class and epoch.

The same thing happens with an oppressed person who is producing images of his own oppression: we must identify with him, sympathetically. *Solidarity will not suffice.* His oppression must be our own.

In order for metaxis to come about, the image must become autonomous. When this is the case, *the image of the real is real as image.*

The oppressed creates *images of his reality.* Then, he must play with *the reality of these images.* The oppressions remain the same, but they are presented in transubstantiated form. The oppressed must forget the real world which was the origin of the image and play with the image itself, in its artistic embodiment. He must make an extrapolation from his social reality towards the reality which is called fiction (towards theatre, towards image) and, having played with the image, he must make a second extrapolation, now in the inverse direction, towards the social reality which is his world. *He practises in the second world (the aesthetic), in order to modify the first (the social).*

This transubstantiation must be effected by the oppressed-artist himself. It is he who must create the image, in whatever form he sees fit, on which the participants are to work.

It is very important to maintain the coherence of this new world that has been created. When playing with the image, no reference should be made back to the world which begot it. Each of the two worlds has its own organic constitution.

The second hypothesis can be formulated thus: if the oppressed-artist is able to create an autonomous world of images of his own reality, and to enact his liberation in the reality of these images, he will then extrapolate into his own life all that he has accomplished in the fiction. The scene, the stage, becomes the rehearsal space for real life.

Third hypothesis: analogical induction

In a Theatre of the Oppressed session where the participants belong to the same social group (students at the same school, residents of the same district, workers at the same factory) and suffer the same oppressions (*vis-à-vis* the school, the district or the factory), the individual account of a single person will immediately be pluralised: so the oppression of one is the oppression of all. The particularity of each individual case is negligible in relation to its similarity with all the others. So, during the session, sympathy is immediate. *We are all talking about ourselves.*

On the other hand, in a specific Cop in the Head or Rainbow of Desire session it may happen that someone tells a story of individual oppression, the details of which can become *singularised* in the extreme, removed from the particular circumstances of the other participants. In such a situation, we will be held in the grip of empathy, we will become spectators of the teller of the story. Even though we may place ourselves in solidarity with that person, this will no longer be the Theatre of the Oppressed, it will only be *theatre for one oppressed.*

The Theatre of the Oppressed is the theatre of the first person plural. It is absolutely vital to begin with an individual account, but if it does not pluralise of its own accord we must go beyond it by means of analogical induction, so that it may be studied by all the participants.

The third hypothesis may be formulated thus: if, setting out from an opening image or scene, one proceeds by analogy to create other images (or scenes) produced by the other participants in the session around their own similar individual oppressions, and if, with these images as the starting point, one arrives by induction at the construction of a model untrammelled by, disengaged from, the singular circumstances of each specific case, this model will contain the general mechanisms by means of which the oppression is produced, which will allow us to study sympathetically the different possibilities for breaking this oppression.

The function of analogical induction is to allow a distanced analysis, to offer several perspectives, to multiply the possible points of view from which one can consider each situation. *We do not interpret, we explain nothing, we only offer multiple points of reference. The oppressed must be helped to reflect on his own action (by looking at alternatives which may be possible, shown to him by other participants who, for their part, are thinking about their own singularities). A disjunction of action and reflection on that action must be brought about.* The protagonist must see himself *qua* protagonist and *qua* object. He is the observer and the person observed.

The validity of these three hypotheses rests on the fundamental hypothesis underlying the totality of the Theatre of the Oppressed: if the oppressed himself performs an action (rather than the artist in his place), the performance of that action in theatrical fiction will enable him to activate himself to perform it in his real life.

This hypothesis expressly contradicts the theory of catharsis, according to which the 'vicarious' attitude of the spectator produces in him a voiding of the emotions which he has experienced during the show.

4 EXPERIENCES IN TWO PSYCHIATRIC HOSPITALS

Sartrouville

Annick Echappasse had warned me: 'There won't be many people, maybe five or six adolescents. One can never be sure, because from time to time they go off on training courses and placements which sometimes lead to full-time jobs. There will also be a trainee, who is following the theatre work we are doing. So, altogether, with the two of us, we will be eight or nine people at the most. The room isn't terribly big, but we manage.'

The first day was a big shock for me. I had seen people who are labelled 'mentally handicapped'⊚ before – I had seen them on the bus, in the street. My entire experience of 'handicapped' people had been with people who had no expectations of me, people who weren't even aware of my presence. Accidental, circumstantial encounters.

⊚ The terms 'learning difficulty', 'mental disability' and so on, which are now more acceptable to the disabled community, were not current when Boal did this work. Also his self-confessed inexperience of this constituency led him, at that time, to conflate acquired mental illness with disability from birth (A.J.).

Sartrouville was the occasion of my first face-to-face meeting with such people with the intention of dialogue, exchange: there were expectations on both sides.

My first impression was utterly superficial. I was struck by their similarity, their tics, their repetitive movements, their difficulty in articulating their *difference*.

Annick kicked off the session:

> 'What do you want to do?'

> 'Nothing,' said one of them.

All were agreed on this point. Annick as well.

> 'Fine. We'll do nothing. With that end in mind, we'll divide into two groups who will each do nothing. Augusto will go off with one group and I'll stay with the other. Each group has to try and do nothing, in their own way. We'll give it about half an hour and then we'll meet back here and show each other that we have done nothing. OK?'

Yes, they were OK about doing nothing . . . in two groups. I went off with my group, the smaller one, the men's group, like a good father. Annick, the good mother, stayed with the women.

> 'So,' I said, 'we're going to try doing nothing. What does anyone suggest by way of starting point?'

'Nothing,' answered Andres.

'Yes, OK, that's already been settled. But how are we going to show this *nothing*? We have to show that we are doing nothing: that has to be clear. For example, if we stay like this, they'll say we're waiting for something: waiting – which is already doing something. We must show them that we're not waiting for anything, that we're doing nothing. How?'

Andres thought quickly.

'Ah, yes, right . . . this is what we do: I lie down on the ground and pretend to be sleeping. . . . And that's it. . . . ' Andres was still doing all the talking.

'OK, you lie down on the ground and pretend to be sleeping. So we've already got something to show them. How do you sleep?'

He showed us how he slept.

'I sleep like this, on the floor. That's all there is to it. . . . '

'Then what?'

'Then nothing. . . . '

'Nothing? But in that case I don't know if you're sleeping or if you're dead or if you're pretending or what. . . . You'll have to do something else. . . . '

Andres gave the matter some thought.

'OK, then you come in, you tap me on the shoulder, but I don't move. I am sleeping, that's all. That's doing nothing. . . . '

He stopped talking and laughed.

'What are you laughing at?' I asked.

'When I sleep, I have dreams. . . . '

'Very well. So that means that you are doing something when you are doing nothing.'

'Yes.'

'When you are doing nothing and sleeping you have dreams. So, you are still doing something. . . . I've got a feeling that it is actually impossible to do nothing at all. . . . We're always doing something.'

'Yes . . . me, I dream.'

'And what do you dream about?'

'Horses.'

'And what else?'

'Just horses. I have dreams with horses . . . that's all.'

'Do you like horses?'

'Yes, I like horses. . . . '

To one side, Georges was watching us. I became aware that I was not talking to Andres alone. Some small progress had already been made. We could change interlocutors so as not to put too much pressure on Andres, not to tire him out.

'What about you, Georges, what do you dream about?'

'The cinema.'

'You dream of being an actor?'

'No.'

'What then?'

'Director.'

'Great. You want to be a film director? Perhaps we could act that out to show the girls.'

'Yes. We could.'

I am by nature verbose; they on the other hand were very direct and straight to the point. I picked up a bit of wood lying on the floor and made as if I had a camera in my hand.

'There you go, Georges: I have a camera in my hand. I can film anything I want. There: I am filming your foot, your arm, your face, I come in closer and I am filming your eye, your nose, I back off and I am filming all of you. . . . There. Now, I am giving you the camera. It's your turn. Your turn to shoot. What are you going to film?'

Georges took the fictive camera and started filming whatever took his fancy. I suggested that he give us some direction: what should we do? He started carrying on just like a real director, while Andres was really keen to play the protagonist. The two of them rehearsed what they wanted to show the girls, the *nothing* they had done.

Annick called us back. We returned to the main space where the girls had been rehearsing. She told us:

'We've also done some "nothings" we'd like to show. Who'll go first?'

Andres, the protagonist in Georges' film, was raring to go and asked if they could start. OK.

'Take it away, Georges!'

Georges lay down on the ground; he was asleep. In his dream, he took up his camera, then gave directions to Andres, the film's protagonist: back a bit, re-shoot the scene that went wrong, shake hands with another member of the cast. Then he moved in, camera in hand, took some close-ups, some mid-shots; he backed away, asked us to smile, to shake hands, to sit down, to stand up. In short, he ordered us about just like a real film director!

I thought his idea was excellent, and so did Annick. She suggested to the other adolescents that they do the same, take the fictive camera and have a go at filming. The enormous mobilising power of the game dawned on us. The principle was simple: with a camera in hand, real or pretend, the individual became a protagonist, an active subject, not an object. Taking hold of a camera, even a pretend camera, meant deciding on an action. Even if that action was showing *nothing*. Even if it was only a dream.

Annick had said: 'Show nothing!' To show this nothing, it was necessary to act, to do something. Put another way, it was necessary to negate the nothing. This requirement found its realisation in the need to use the camera.

Most of the adolescents willingly took the camera and used it as they saw fit, in line with their own personality – with their own individual stamp.

From this point on it was easier to spot the differences between them. My first impression had been: 'They are all mentally handicapped.' A generalisation: they're all the same. Now, everyone was showing much more of themselves, their nuances, their individuality. They were 'handicapped', sure, but they were not *madmen*.

Each of them impressed me in his or her own way. Especially Georges, who wanted to be a film director and had had the excellent idea of playing with a camera. The session over, Annick and I went off together. In the car, I admitted to her that I was astonished. I told her everything, from my first impressions to my final impression. And I said to her:

> 'You know, Annick, that guy, Georges. . . . He didn't seem in the
> least bit handicapped or ill. I'd even go so far as to say that he struck
> me as very intelligent.'

> 'Sure. . . . He's the trainee I was telling you about.'

I had forgotten there was a trainee.

I began to think about it: why forget such a thing? I had said to myself: 'I am going to work with some mentally handicapped people.' With that starting point, I had begun to prepare myself for a dialogue with *handicapped people*. I began to see handicapped people everywhere. From the moment I entered that medico-professional environment, everyone, for me, was a potential handicapped person. Even the director of the establishment, a very courteous man, only escaped such consideration because he was over forty and I knew that the department only accepted patients under twenty. But several other younger teachers had struck me as a little strange . . . lugubrious, even. In short, mad.

In reality, it was not that difficult to think of all these people as mentally handicapped: everyone has some nervous tic or other, everyone has a *different* look about them, everyone walks in a way which is *not normal*. Isn't that so? You and me, for instance.

Question: what is normal?

The mechanism is very simple: from the moment I was told 'they are mentally handicapped', I took them for mentally handicapped people. Anyone who presented themselves to my sight would have been welcomed with the same kindness (with a hint of pity, of commiseration).

From then on, I started observing the behaviour of the other teachers or care workers towards the adolescents. And I noticed similarities. With two differences – first, they knew very well and so could easily distinguish who was *sick* and who was *of sound mind*, except in the case of a new arrival (me, for example – had I been younger I would have run a serious risk of classification in the former category); second, in front of the patients, they did not come across as particularly *kind*, rather they seemed *forceful.*

I used especially to watch the care workers who came into a big room where I would wait at the start of each session; within the one room there were lots of people: adolescents, members of staff and so on. The care workers would come in and it was fascinating to watch their faces, the changes in their physiognomy according to who they were looking at. When their eyes fell on me, they were courtesy itself, but the moment their eyes fell on a young person they acquired authority, an aspect of forcefulness.

Suppose that, like Georges, I had been taken for a patient. How long would I have been able to resist? Not all my life. Once saddled with the image of madman, how would one convince people that it was not true? How could one avoid accommodating oneself to this image? It would have been difficult for me, but even more so for a young person.

I am not for a moment suggesting that these adolescents became ill as a result of the way other people looked at them. Not at all. Much further back in time, they had their families. And many of them had had alcoholic parents, miserable childhoods, had grown up in bad neighbourhoods, with drugs, physical violence, assault, promiscuity and the whole usual catalogue of misfortunes. It had taken more than a mere stare for them to end up where they had.

But I was powerfully struck by the way people looked. Because I had done it myself.

Fleury-les-Aubrais

At the invitation of Dr Roger Gentis, Cecilia Thumim and I led a Theatre of the Oppressed workshop twice a week at Fleury-les-Aubrais psychiatric hospital, over a period of two months. We had thirty trainees: nurses, doctors and members of the hospital's administrative staff.

Claude, a nurse, was the first to propose a theme and a story for the Forum Theatre models. He told us how one Sunday afternoon when he was on duty, a Yugoslav arrived at the hospital. He had broken some bottles at the local bistro, knocked over tables, hurt a few people. His football team had lost, and the poor man had had a violent fit. To cap it all, the Yugoslav didn't speak a word of French. Correction: he knew how to say 'Pas de piqure! Pas de piqure!'⊚ It wasn't much, to be sure, but enough to forearm him against needles.

⊚ 'No injections, no injections.'

The patient was shut up in a veritable cell of a hospital room, and a doctor, having carried out a summary examination, prescribed him a tranquilliser . . . to be delivered intramuscularly. Claude had the task of performing this dosage. He went into the cell, telling the patient: 'This won't hurt.' As you might imagine, the reply he received was: 'Pas de piqure! Pas de piqure!' And the Yugoslav cowered at the back of the cell.

Claude persisted, but the response was a total and vehement refusal: 'Pas de piqure! Pas de piqure!' There was nothing to be done. Claude locked the cell door, and went back to the doctor's room; but he too was unbending:

> 'I am the doctor here. My duty is to prescribe medication. You are a nurse and your duty is to carry out my orders. Go back in there and do the injection!'

Claude went back into the ward, solicited the help of four of his more burly friends, and they set off, like 'brothers in arms'. They swept into the cell, grabbed hold of the Yugoslav cringing in his corner, threw him face down on the bed, and ignoring his supplications – 'Pas de piqure! Pas de piqure!' – gave him the prescribed injection; they were in the grip of such a fury that they might well have done far worse to him.

While he was telling the story, Claude was euphoric, overexcited. At the end, he became sad:

> 'What could I do? I wasn't the doctor. If I had said no, he could have had me demoted, he could have got in the way of my promotion, put in a report against me. He said he was the person in charge and that was true; he was the person in charge . . . but I was the one who did it. I did the injection because I need my job and I could see no way round it.

But I felt guilty when I looked at the guy after the injection . . . he was holding back his tears . . . it was ghastly . . . but what would you have done in my place?'

That is Forum Theatre in a nutshell: what would we have done? So we prepared the model: the arrival of the Yugoslav, the doctor's orders, the first refusal, the return to the doctor's office, the search for muscular allies; finally, the denouement.

Claude asked us to make the Forum Theatre show public: we had to announce it to the whole hospital complex (which comprised about ten buildings, including a restaurant and the administration department) and invite the whole staff: the doctors and especially the nurses. Claude wanted to know what others would have done in his place. The announcement was made, with entirely predictable consequences – which none of us had predicted: the patients heard about the show and wanted to see it.

Panic ! We had anticipated an internal forum, we were already facing a potential minor multitude, and now . . . the patients. Would it be right to let them in? They featured in the play, sure, but in the form of a pretext, part of the scenario. Would it be right to let them take part in discussions, debates, exchanges of ideas, of which they were the 'object'?

The 'yesses' were in the majority. The Theatre of the Oppressed being a democratic form of theatre (which is absolutely the case!) we could not refuse entry to the patients. They came, with enthusiasm . . . and in numbers: they formed at least 80 per cent of the audience.

To be honest, I was scared. It was the first time I had seen such an audience. What should I say? How should I explain? Don't forget that I am no therapist; I am a man of the theatre. I had had to confront difficult audiences in the past – if this one seemed to me even more difficult, it was precisely because I had no desire to 'confront' it, nor could I have done so. I could not 'direct' it, nor did I wish to. This was my great quandary: how to establish a rapport with the audience? In thirty-five years of professional theatre, I had learnt a thousand different ways to address the *animateur*–audience relationship. But here, it was all new to me.

Cecilia suggested that I should behave just as I would in a normal situation. So I decided to change nothing, to act as I always do, whatever the Forum Theatre show. And this is what I did. I explained the rules of the game. I offered a few exercises, ones which have always proved most effective whatever the nature of the audience. And I observed that the patients did them better than the staff. I said this to Claude, who countered:

'True, but that's because they are concentrating on the exercise, while we are busy concentrating on them.'

Once a state of theatrical communion had been established, we started to perform the model.

It was wonderful to behold. For the first time, patients were present at discussions of which they were the object; for the first time, they were present at conferences between doctors and nurses, they saw 'how the other half lives', they discovered what people thought of them, which was, generally speaking, very different from what was said to their faces. It was wonderful. And it became more and more moving.

The model finished. I repeated the rules of the game: anyone who wanted to intervene to try an alternative only had to say 'Stop!' The actors would interrupt the action, the spect-actor would replace the protagonist and the improvisation would begin.

We started again. In the audience, silence; a tense silence, in contrast to the hilarity which had greeted the showing of the model. Then, the patients had been laughing and having fun; now, they were assuming a responsibility: it was they who were being questioned. People wanted to know what they thought. Silence. First sequence, second sequence . . . finally, the Claude character (who was none other than the man himself) made his first threat to carry out the injection. Silence. The Yugoslav does not want an injection. He gives vent to his habitual cry, 'Pas de piqure! Pas de piqure!'

'Stop!'

It is Robert, a strange patient, with a veritable repertoire of nervous tics, who I was used to seeing sneaking round the gardens, creeping behind trees. He interrupts the scene.

We stop. Robert stands up and approaches the improvised stage. I ask him, in a tone which in spite of myself comes out as paternal:

'Have you got the idea, Robert? You have to show what you think Claude should have done, what you would have done in his place. Do you understand, Robert? Is it clear?'

'It's clear enough. . . .'

Claude takes off his white coat and gives it to Robert, who enjoys handling it. Like a real actor, he is experiencing the pleasure of dressing up in the character's costume, getting into role, thinking of himself as a nurse. In a moment, he will be the nurse. He enters the scene, while I, unable to shake off my paternalist tone, warn him again:

'Robert, show what Claude should have done!'

The scene takes up again from where it has been stopped: at the moment when the actor playing the Yugoslav protests: 'Pas de piqure! Pas de piqure!' the only thing he knows how to say. 'What?' asked Robert. 'Explain a bit better. What do you mean?' The actor-Yugoslav, in reality a young woman doctor, improvises a foreign language, muttering a fictive Serbo-Croat. Understanding nothing, Robert goes to the table, takes the telephone, dials a hypothetical number, and asks:

'Is that the Yugoslav embassy? Please, send a translator over to the hospital as a matter of urgency, we have one of your compatriots here who is going on and on about something, but we can't understand a bloody word . . . .'

The audience was moved. Such a simple solution could only have been found by a 'sick person'. We, the 'healthy', had not thought of it. Robert, delighted with the effect of his intervention, explained:

'What if, in his own language, he was trying to say that he could not have injections because of an allergy? The injection could have killed the poor man.'

The Serbo-Croat language was incomprehensible to us. We did not speak Serbo-Croat. But that was no reason not to hear what he had to say. And, to hear what he had to say, we needed a translator.

Many other alternatives were presented that evening. Not all pleased the spectators, 'sick' or 'healthy': for instance, another 'sick person', who won the Yugoslav's confidence by distracting his attention with a football and then, treacherously, gave him the injection. Many 'sick' and 'healthy' people took turns in the search for viable solutions. The last was a patient who had been 'sectioned', confined by order of the courts, a woman of about fifty, morose, sad, taciturn; on meeting the Yugoslav's refusal, the 'Pas de piqure!', she kissed her white coat goodbye with:

'He doesn't want the injection . . . I am not giving it.'

And she left the stage without waiting for the applause that followed. She went back to her chair and stayed there, taciturn, sad and morose; one 'sick person' who had just reminded us of the dignity of another 'sick person', the Yugoslav. The reduced condition of his health did not rob him of his essential human dignity:

> 'He doesn't want it, I won't do it to him! He is a man. He exists, so he has a right to say no. And we have a duty to respect that.'

5 PRELIMINARIES TO THE UTILISATION OF THE RAINBOW OF DESIRE TECHNIQUES

1 The modes

The techniques presented in this book can all be used in a variety of different ways. The *mode* is an auxiliary technique which can be used as a complement to another technique, to add depth to the exploration being undertaken and to facilitate the discovery and comprehension of a scene and the relations between its characters.[◉] A single technique can be realised in distinct and diverse modes, each with its own specific utility and its own particular properties.

◉ Several of these modes are detailed in greater length, with slightly different applications, in *Games for Actors and Non-Actors*, London: Routledge, 1992.

THE 'NORMAL' MODE

The normal mode is the real base on which an improvisation is built. I say real and not realistic, since realistic is a word over-charged with connotations of theatrical style. The goal to be aimed for in improvisation is reality, not realism. The protagonist and the other actors must aim for truth rather than likelihood, verity rather than verisimilitude. An improvisation can be real even if it is surrealistic, expressionistic, symbolic, metaphorical, allegorical. An improvisation is real when it is *lived*.

Before the start of an improvisation in the normal mode, which usually serves as a base for all the work, the person who is leading must make sure – and I lay great stress on this point – that the structure is sufficiently theatrical. Then the improvisation unfolds; its point of departure, its moment of crisis and even its denouement can be known in advance without one knowing in what manner the action will unfold, what its characteristics will be – that is where the improvisation comes in. All improvisation is a quest, a process of discovery. In order for that quest to be effective, the structure of the scene from which it sets out needs to be as dynamic as possible.

For this reason, the person leading must ensure that each actor *knows what their character wants*. By this I mean that each actor must be directed to *live* the *desire* of their character intensely, rather than merely exhibiting that desire on the stage. As long as each character has an intense desire, as long as he or she intensely desires something – or does not desire something, which is also a form of desire, a negative desire – these desires will inevitably enter into conflict and from this conflict will spring the dramatic action. Theatre is conflict, not the mere exhibition of states of mind.

If the 'wills'[⊚] mobilising the characters are essential wills – intense desires, wills which relate to the real necessities of these characters and not to their caprices – the dramatic action will wend its way towards a crisis, where a choice will have to be made. The *point of crisis* must come across as the moment at which a structure of human relations has developed to a point where different alternatives to what follows are possible. That's why in the Theatre of the Oppressed we refer to *Chinese crisis*: in Chinese, there is no single ideogram for the word 'crisis', which is instead expressed by two ideograms, one meaning 'danger' and the other 'opportunities'. The collision of these two meanings defines 'crisis' in its usage in Theatre of the Oppressed terminology.

⊚ For more on Boal's use of 'wills' and 'counter-wills' see *Games for Actors and Non-Actors*, pp. 51–9.

Generally speaking, in improvisations based on actual facts from the life of the protagonists, when the latter arrive at a point of crisis, they choose the alternative which suits them least, or the undesired alternative whose consequences they regret. Usually it is in this nucleus, in this hotbed of conflict, that the most important elements of the structure of relations between the characters are to be found. It is therefore this point of crisis which must be studied, analysed, intensified.

In order to reach a Chinese crisis, the characters' wills, their desires and ambitions, must be very intense. Theatre is conflict, for the simple reason that life is conflict. Theatre is life, and life is theatre.

THE 'BREAKING THE OPPRESSION' MODE

Often, participants will tell stories and suggest improvisations in which the protagonist is extremely weak, resigned, bereft of desires. This generally arises from the fact that the actual scene 'has already taken place' in real life. And although everything that has already taken place 'continues to take place' (with differing degrees of intensity according to the emotional importance of the event experienced) the protagonist has often almost given up: 'That's how it is, there is nothing to be done.'

If there really is nothing to be done, it is not even worth trying. But usually something can be done. Experience shows that the protagonist, in the simple act of recounting the scene she experienced or proposing to make an improvisation out of it, is revealing her desire to relive it, to transform it, to examine its variations and alternatives. So, we must try.

Sometimes the initial improvisation may turn out to be too flimsy, too weak, lacking in power and interest. When this is the case, the improvisation needs to be reworked to enable and encourage subsequent intervention by the other participants and to give the protagonist herself the opportunity to recharge her own desire to transform the scene and to try other alternatives. It is frequently the case that in the first improvisation, the protagonist does not reveal what is really essential to her.

It should be noted that, faced with a conflict which is too weak and uninteresting, our creativity will not be stimulated. One could draw an analogy with attending a boxing match in which one of the boxers enters the ring on crutches, limping – clearly such a match would not interest us, since its outcome would be predictable, even before the first punch had been thrown. So it is with theatre, with improvisation. The protagonist must have some possibilities of victory. If, however, on account of her innate weakness or the extreme disparity of the forces in conflict, the protagonist is inexorably doomed to failure, let us not be masochists: let us not use theatre to work on a scene which will lead us unerringly to despair.

The breaking the oppression mode essentially consists of asking the protagonist to relive the scene not as it really happened, but as it could have happened or could happen in the future – the way she would like it to happen. The protagonist is instructed to try even harder than she did in the original scene to overcome the oppression facing her. The antagonists, of course, do not remain inert, they react with a corresponding increase of determination, and the temperature of the whole conflict tends to rise. The dynamic having been restored, the situation becomes clearer and the alternatives more evident.

The breaking the oppression mode can help this process of dramatisation and clarification, but it is sometimes insufficient because at times the protagonist herself does not know, does not recognise, or quite simply cannot see, certain essential elements of the scene. In this latter case, we use the 'Stop and think!' mode.

THE 'STOP AND THINK!' MODE

This is a rehearsal technique which I have used for many years in the course of rehearsals for shows in the so-called 'normal' professional theatre.

This mode is predicated on the fact that just as we cannot prevent our hearts from beating or our lungs from respiring, similarly we cannot stop our brain from thinking. Our senses function without cease: we constantly perceive what we touch, we continually smell the odours that we breathe, our ears never stop hearing, our palates detect tastes, and even with closed lids, our eyes still see through the eyes of the memory, our mind's eye.

These sensations, present or memorised, affect us ceaselessly, with variable intensities, and sometimes imperceptibly. They make us think and we think at lightning speed. We have hundreds of thoughts per second; thought is swift and indomitable. Of course, we do not have the capacity to translate all these thoughts into words. A word occupies time and space. It takes time to pronounce a word, even if the word is not spoken out loud but only mentally articulated, with closed mouth. Sometimes a fraction of a second is long enough for us to have an idea – 'I have an idea' – and the idea is there, whole, complete, with ramifications, complex. But if someone asked us to expound this idea which came in a flash, it would take us a long time to explain it. Thought flies at the speed of light, but its enunciation, its articulation in words comprehensible to the interlocutor, plods along like a horse and cart.

So we think light and we talk matter. For that reason, much light remains without flesh: almost nothing of what we think is expressed. Millions of our thoughts are never spoken.

This mode is relatively simple: once the improvisation is properly in gear, the director says 'Stop!' whenever she suspects that a gesture is shielding something hidden. The actors must then freeze their movements in mid-action. If an actor is caught in the act of walking, his foot in mid-air, he must stay like that. If another is stretching out his hand towards a third, their hands not yet touching, they must not touch. If the 'Stop!' surprises an actor looking at something he particularly wanted to avoid looking at, he must keep looking. And all the actors stay motionless. The director then says: 'Think!' Still motionless, without any kind of censorship or self-censorship, they must all speak out loud everything in their minds as the character, without stopping, transforming into words all the thoughts that come into their heads. Without censorship or self-censorship, they must allow their 'body' – not only their brains but every part of their body – to think of its position in space and also of this position in relation to the other bodies, the other people and objects.

After a bit, the director says: 'Action!' and the actors take up the improvisation exactly where they left off when interrupted. In this exercise the actors need not attempt to hear what their colleagues are saying; all of them are to vocalise only their 'interior monologue' – no dialogue is allowed.

In the absence of movement, there is the opportunity for the utterance of all unexpressed thoughts; similarly, fugitive or taboo thoughts can more easily come to light. And we discover things that were ready to come out, things we were unaware of thinking, but that were, none the less, thoughts, sensations, emotions, with potential consequences, for better or for worse. We should be aware that any unexpressed thought, emotion or sensation will always, inevitably, find issue in other unconscious, invisible ways.

This mode helps to make conscious, to verbalise and thus transmit, to make comprehensible, the hidden, the diluted, the hitherto imperceptible.

THE 'SOFTLY SOFTLY' MODE – SLOW AND LOW

Sometimes a scene gets too violent – emotions that have not as yet exploded in real life, explode here and now! The actors playing such a situation have a tendency to be less creative, no longer to improvise in depth, but to expend all their energies in shouting and physical force, in contortions and tensions confined to the musculature. At such times it is advisable for the director to propose the softly softly mode: after several minutes of a normal, but violent improvisation – it should not be forgotten that violence can 'charge up' actors – the director asks the actors to speak as quietly as possible for the rest of the improvisation, in barely audible voices, as slowly and as clearly as possible. Their movements must also be very slow; they must move in slow motion.

By speaking so quietly and moving so slowly, the actors acquire an enhanced power of self-observation, they become more attentive spectators of themselves and their actions. Because of the slowness, each gesture appears magnified; by their secretive tone, the words reveal their true content.

The softly softly mode can be used during the working process of any Theatre of the Oppressed technique, particularly after use of the normal mode, if the latter becomes too aggressive or too crude. Equally it is an integral part of a technique we will be developing later on (the Image of the Antagonist, see p. 118). It is also a mode which I currently use in rehearsals for conventional theatre shows; it restores the sensitivity of skin-deep actors and allows them to perceive with greater acuity their relations with the other characters.

THE 'LIGHTNING FORUM' MODE

When a session of Forum Theatre is under way, the spect-actor has the right to interrupt the action to try her alternative. To do this, she needs time and space. And she must be given all the time and space she needs, she must be assured of total tranquillity so that she may apply her tactic or strategy to the best of her ability. In Forum Theatre the intention is to verify each alternative in depth.

However, in the Rainbow of Desire work process, the forum format can on occasion be used not for the detailed analysis of each intervention, but as a way of providing the protagonist with a palette of possibilities, even if these possibilities are only sketched out, enunciated or envisaged. In Forum Theatre proper, where the important thing is to be able to analyse the situation presented, to study it objectively, it is vital that each intervention be enacted in complete freedom and complete safety. With Rainbow of Desire techniques, however, though the situation itself is still important, the protagonist is more important. Here it is not a matter of verifying 'what *we* could do in such a situation' but 'what *the protagonist* can do, if he is capable of it, in a situation like this'. In shifting the centre of attention from the situation to the protagonist, the lightning forum mode has the virtue of offering the latter a whole gamut of suggestions: 'What if you tried something a bit like this?' The very imprecision of the proposition allows the protagonist later to adapt it to his actual possibilities.

The lightning forum mode consists of a high-speed forum, a forum at a run. To achieve this, the director can even line up the participants, and send them on stage one by one in front of the protagonist, who observes each improvisation. In turn, they take the protagonist's place on stage. Each spends just enough time there, a minute or two at most, to try out their alternative in a condensed but intense fashion. The director limits the time given to each as he sees fit and then sends the next person on stage to take over, without letting the improvisation come to a halt. This means that the antagonist carries on with his action right till the last actor has tried his suggestion or the real protagonist gets back in position.

THE 'AGORA' MODE

The agora mode verifies the internal forces acting on the protagonist during his moments of rest; not the forces at work in the action itself – the action of the conflict(s) with other characters – but those at work when he is in conflict with himself.

Whenever possible, when using any technique which, broadly speaking, analyses and deconstructs the elements of the will or desire of the protagonist – such as the specific technique called Rainbow of Desire – it is advisable to end the session with the agora mode. This consists of bringing the protagonist out of the scene and asking the other characters who are impersonating the protagonist's desires to engage in dialogue and in actions with each other.

The agora mode can also be used when several antagonists are in place. In such a case, we exclude the protagonist and it is the antagonists who enter into conflict with each other, become allies, create new structures.

THE 'FAIR' MODE

The most useful feature of the fair mode is that it liberates the actors from the excessive pressure generated by the audience which, even if one thinks of it as a group of spect-actors, does have a physical presence. There is a danger of actors tensing up when observed by an audience, when a whole audience is concentrated on the observation of a single action. This is the time to introduce the fair mode: a number of improvisations are presented simultaneously around the room, like stalls at a fair, allowing the actors to concentrate exclusively on the one they are part of. The clamour of a roomful of improvisations has some stimulating effects and can enhance the creativity of each individual actor. Paradoxically, the multiplication of movement and sound can sometimes aid concentration instead of interfering with it.

For the actor, concentration is not a matter of putting oneself into a nirvana-like state, a state of nothingness. For actors, concentrating means endowing themselves with the capacity intensely to direct their attention and their powers of perception towards those things that really matter to them in the scene, the things they come into contact with, interact with. If such a 'thing' is another actor, concentration means establishing an intense interrelationship with this other, speaking and listening, seeing and being seen, giving and receiving.

THE 'THREE WISHES' MODE

It is possible that on observing a scene, a situation, after the fleeting moment of its enactment, we may not arrive at an understanding of what the protagonist really wants, which stops us from helping her, from imagining – and offering – alternatives for her.

The three wishes mode can unblock the situation. The director gets the participants to transform the scene into a frozen image. He gives the protagonist the right to make three wishes come true. 'First wish: action!' Ten seconds later: 'Stop!' And so on, three times. On each wish, the protagonist is allowed to modify the image of the scene substantially, without the other actors either hindering or helping her. The protagonist must bring about whatever modification she considers necessary or desirable, on her own.

In this mode, the protagonist sculpts her wishes herself, by manipulating the image, by physically changing it and, by the same token, changing herself.

Sometimes, after the first series of three wishes, I offer the protagonist three more wishes; and then another three. It is a curious thing: almost always, the protagonist wearies of wishing, or chooses to stop at the third or fourth wish, thus revealing that her overriding wish or desire was to eliminate what she did not desire, to do away with what was troubling her, without, for all that, wishing to create anything else in its place.

Frequently, at the end of the technique, I offer the protagonist the opportunity to stage a last wish, but for this I let her have as much time as she needs to follow the wish through to its very end. Generally, she answers: 'It'll take too long', as if humanity was not prepared to realise its desires, as if the state of desiring was the most we could hope for. As if it was best not to make the first wish come true, since after that there will still be a second wish, and a third, and the ultimate wish. And yet our life is, of necessity, permanently composed of desire, will, want, need – even if our only desire is to desire. Do I desire something, or do I just desire desire?

THE 'DISSOCIATION' MODE

Sometimes the content of a scene can suggest that there is a discrepancy between the characters' declared desires and their inner wishes. This mode consists of separating the *interior monologue* from the *exterior dialogue* and from the *desire in action*. First, the actors in the image are asked to verbalise, over several minutes, the thoughts which assail them, while keeping the image immobile and rigid. Then they are asked to engage in dialogue, to whatever extent they are able to, still without moving. Finally they must try to show, by means of a mute physical action, their desires converted into reality, in the form of the image in motion. Their desires are expressed by the movement of their bodies.

THE 'PLAYING TO THE DEAF' MODE

This technique is particularly useful when a scene appears over-dependent on words, at the expense of action or physical expression; in these cases, it often feels as if the scene would work just as well as radio drama. In 'playing to the deaf', the actors rerun the improvisation of a scene, this time attempting to make it as clear as possible as if for a deaf public. The gestures become more significant, denser, stronger. Without the prop of words, the actors attempt to communicate through the senses everything that was previously expressed verbally – by the way they use their bodies, by their movements, by objects they use and the way they use them, by the duration of their actions. When we cannot use words our bodies become much more expressive.

2 The improvisation

Most of the Rainbow of Desire techniques start with an improvisation. The complexity and richness of the image work which follows depend on the complexity and richness of this first improvisation. To develop this vital first step as fully as possible, there are a number of precautions the director should take:

1 The protagonist must choose each participant herself; the director must not allow her just to address a request to everyone in general: 'Two men, two women.' No! It is up to the protagonist to choose which men and which women. A director can already perceive many things from the very process of this choice: which actors have been chosen, but also which have not been chosen; was the choice made quickly or did it take time? Did the protagonist vacillate between two of the actors? Did she go back to her first choice? Did she choose a woman to play a man? Why? During this process of choosing, the protagonist's body moves, and this movement is in itself a writing. This writing can and must be read.

2 The protagonist must exercise the functions of dramaturg and director: she must compose the scenario, point out the conflicts and the psychological characteristics of the characters, and suggest the main movements – the markers – of the scene. The actors must follow all the protagonist's directions to the letter.

3 If the improvisation turns out to be theatrically impoverished (for example, a bunch of actors sitting opposite each other around a table) the director must – in maieutic fashion – pose a lot of questions: on the location of the action and its surroundings; on the characters' movements, their habits, the way they live, their occupations. Their movements are especially important. What do the characters do while they're talking? Do they move about? What about while they're working? When and how do they enjoy themselves? It is often in movements that the rituals of oppression are most embedded. For that reason, whenever possible the director should ask the characters to enter a scene, rather than starting the improvisation with

them already installed on stage. The entry into the scene is, likewise, a writing.

In order to enrich the initial improvisation with detail, the director can also ask the actors and the protagonist to rehearse the scene in the 'playing to the deaf' mode, that is, rehearsing without words. This type of rehearsal, because it magnifies gestures, movements and facial expressions, can make both characters and scene more eloquent.

4 Above all the director must insist on each person knowing clearly what their character *wants*. Theatre is conflict, action. It is not enough for the actor merely to display, she must do something, she must act. The actor is a verb, not an adjective. Romeo is a man who loves a woman; he is not winged love, nor is he just a face with love written all over it. What is each person's will? This is absolutely essential, even when this will is to want nothing.

3 Identification, recognition and resonance

Several of the techniques presented in the second part of this book involve the construction of images, sometimes by the protagonist, sometimes by the other participants.

In order to be able to dynamise a complex of images, the actors who are to animate them must have strong, intense feelings in relation to them. The director must verify the nature of this relationship. Bearing in mind the objectives of the work, it is my belief that only three types of relationship between actor and image will lead to fruitful and creative results.

IDENTIFICATION

We can use the term 'identification' when the actor is able to say: 'I am exactly like that.' Identification is the strongest of these three types of actor–image relation, since it is the actor's own personality which animates it, her own sensibility, rather than just the approximate knowledge she may have of another person's sensibility.

RECOGNITION

'I am not like that at all, but I know exactly the sort of person it's talking about!' In this case, the actor will be mobilised by her knowledge of an 'other', by real-life experiences she has had with an 'other'; she will be mobilised not because the image relates directly to her but because it relates to this 'other', whom she knows well. This relationship will be that much more intense if the actor has experienced or is still experiencing a relationship of opposition to the image (or the character) which she claims to know or recognise.

RESONANCE

Resonance is the most diffuse, but not the least, of these three types of actor–image relation. Resonance is extremely useful for certain techniques which particularly explore aleatory, incidental relations, and which engage in a kind of 'random' research. This form of relation can be said to exist when the image or the character awaken in the actor feelings and emotions which she can only vaguely identify or delineate. 'She is like that, but she could be different'; 'I am not like that, but I would like to be'; 'She could be worse'; 'I don't know, but I have a feeling', and so on.

These three sorts of interrelation will be more effective the more intense they are. Identification is neither more nor less important than resonance, nor is either more or less important than recognition. All three are useful and all three will produce results and discoveries according to their intensity and their richness, and also according to the passion with which the actor commits herself to the image or character and its animation.

4 The four catharses

We speak of catharsis as if all its forms were the same. However, differences exist, are important and can even work in opposition to each other.

Whatever the form, catharsis (from the Greek: κάθαρσις) means purgation, purification, cleaning out. There lies the one and only major similarity between the different forms: the individual or group purifies itself of some element or other which is disturbing its internal equilibrium. The purging of an agent of disturbance is the one element common to all cathartic phenomena.

The differences reside in the nature of what is purged, eliminated. For me, four principal forms of catharsis exist: a medical form, an Aristotelian form, the form used by Moreno, and that used by the Theatre of the Oppressed (including the Cop in the Head techniques, of which catharsis is an integral part).

MEDICAL CATHARSIS

The medical catharsis seeks to eliminate the elements or causes of physical, psychological or psychosomatic suffering of individuals. It works by expelling any element or substance which has introduced itself into the human body or which the body is secreting. That is, it seeks to eliminate something which has its origins within or outside the individual, and which produces in him a sickness. For example, if I eat something unhealthy, or if I take poison, a purgative will result in the expulsion of this noxious element and my health will be restored. For each malady, we seek the relevant medicine or antidote to eliminate it, thus purifying our bodies and soothing our souls.

Apart from tragic catharsis, Aristotle also spoke of 'rhythmic catharsis': the doctor had to discover the 'rhythm' of his patient's mental illness and then induce the patient to sing and dance to this rhythm, as rendered by musical instruments. It was believed that this rhythmic paroxysm would expel the disordered psychic rhythms, leading the patient back to equilibrium and repose.

Medical catharsis could thus act on the physical (notably through purgatives) and the psychological (in the Greek rhythmic catharsis, and in the catharsis defined by Moreno).

'MORENIAN' CATHARSIS

Moreno defined his particular usage of catharsis very well in the famous *Case of Barbara*. Barbara, an actress with an irascible and violent character, could not control the hatred and violence that rose up in her, offstage. Her relationships with others – including and especially her husband – were very difficult, and going from bad to worse. Barbara was an actress in Moreno's troupe. One day, she had to play a violent and irascible prostitute. The act of playing such a character – in one respect identical to herself – purified her of the violence and hatred that were causing her suffering. And this allowed her to adapt to her social life, which was what she had wanted but until then had found impossible to achieve.

In the 'Morenian' catharsis, what is expelled is, in a kind of way, a poison. We can say that its goal is the happiness of the individual (in this exemplary case, that of Barbara and her nearest and dearest).

ARISTOTELIAN CATHARSIS

The Aristotelian catharsis is tragic catharsis. As shown by my study of it in *The Theatre of the Oppressed*, it is a coercive theatrical form. The members of the audience of the Greek tragedy (as with the audience of the Hollywood western, for that matter) go through a process which begins with the exaltation of their own tragic faults (*hamartia*, in Greek), coincident with those of the protagonist, the hero. Then comes the *peripeteia* – the mutation of the happiness caused by this initial exaltation (Oedipus becomes king, Bonnie and Clyde successfully rob banks) into unhappiness (Oedipus discovers his destiny, Bonnie and Clyde have dealings with the police). This process ends with the confession of the faults (*anagnorisis*), empathically assimilated by the spectators, who are also doing their own 'mea culpa', and the *catastrophe* (Oedipus' blinding, the death of Bonnie and Clyde).

In Aristotelian catharsis, what is being eliminated is always the hero's tendency to violate the law, whether human or divine. At the outset, Antigone affirms the rights of the family over the law and over the rights of the state. Oedipus affirms the power of defying fate, *moira*. In the classic westerns, the unhappy Indians or Mexicans affirm the possibility of contravening General Custer's law. And what happens to all of these people? They fall! The spectators are afraid, and submit to catharsis. They purify themselves of their desire for transformation since, in the fiction of the performance, they have already experienced that transformation.

This form of theatrical production – disempowering and tranquillising – seeks, by means of catharsis, to adapt the individual to society. For those who are happy with the values of that society, obviously this form of catharsis is useful. But are we always happy with all of society's values?

CATHARSIS IN THE THEATRE OF THE OPPRESSED

In conventional forms of theatre, the actors' (or characters') action is observed by spectators. In a Theatre of the Oppressed show, spectators do not exist in the simple '*spectare* = to see' sense; here to be a spectator means to be a participant, intervening; here to be a spectator means to prepare oneself for action, and *preparing oneself* is already in itself an action.

In the conventional theatre, there is a code: the code of non-interference by the audience. In the Theatre of the Oppressed, there is a proposition: interference, intervention. In the conventional theatre we present images of the world for contemplation; in the Theatre of the Oppressed, these images are presented to be destroyed and replaced by others. In the first case, the dramatic action is a 'fictitious' action, which substitutes for 'real' action; in the second, the action shown on stage is a possibility, an alternative, and the intervener-spectators (active observers) are called upon to create new actions, new alternatives which are not substitutes for real action, but rehearsals, pre-actions which precede – rather than stand in for – the actual action, the action we want to transform a reality we are trying to change. The rehearsal of an action is in itself an action, the practice of an action then to be practised in real life.

In the conventional theatrical relationship, the actor acts in my place but not in my name. In a Theatre of the Oppressed show anyone can intervene. Not intervening is already a form of intervention: I *decide* to go on stage, but I can also *decide* not to; it is I who choose. The people who do go on stage to try their alternatives go there *in my name* and not *in my place*, because, symbolically, I am there with them. I am – just as they are – a spectator of a new kind: spect-actor. I see and I act.

The goal of the Theatre of the Oppressed is not then to create calm, equilibrium, but rather to create disequilibrium which prepares the way for action. Its goal is to *dynamise*. This dynamisation, with the action which results from it (set off by one spect-actor in the name of all), destroys all the blocks which prohibited the realisation of actions such as this. That is, it purifies the spect-actors, it produces a catharsis. The catharsis of detrimental blocks!

And very welcome it is too!

Part Two | The Practice

1 THE PROSPECTIVE TECHNIQUES

1 The image of the images

Work with a new group should open with this technique. The image of the images can also be used for periodic evaluations of a group. It establishes a relationship between individual, singular problems and the collective problems a group is experiencing.

Stage one: the individual images

The participants form groups of four or five people. Each member of these groups must, in a short space of time, make an image of an actual oppression (one that is still going on at the time, or that could happen again). This image can be realistic, allegorical or surrealistic, it can be symbolic or metaphorical. The only thing that matters is that it is true, that it is felt as true by the protagonist.

The protagonist sculpts the image and then takes up his place in the image, that is, his position as the oppressed. He is not allowed to speak during the construction of the image. To make himself understood by others, the protagonist can use *mirror language*, himself making the gesture or facial expression he wants to see reproduced, or *the language of modelling*, manipulating the actor with his hands, like a sculptor with a statue. The interdiction of words is necessary to enable all the participants to really see the image. Image is a language; if it is translated into words, all its possible interpretations are reduced to a single one: the polysemy of the image is destroyed. But it is precisely in this polysemy that the richness of this language resides.

The protagonist must take up his own position of the oppressed in the image. He puts the other participants in whatever positions he wants, either as oppressors or as allies.

During this first stage, one by one, each of the four or five members of each small group constructs their own individual image, while those who have already been modelled try not to influence the image.

Stage two: the parade of the images

In the second stage, the large group assembles, and each little group, in turn, goes on stage, into the *aesthetic space*. They re-make each of the images in front of everyone.

For each image, the director asks the watching group for objective commentaries. Subjective commentaries can also be expressed, but the director must underline that these are only individual perceptions – feelings, memories, sensations evoked by the image – which must not be taken as definitive *interpretations*. If, in the image presented, a person is seated or standing, that is an objective fact, which could be perceived in different subjective manners. This is why the director must make a distinction between observations of the 'I see this or that' type (things which anybody can see) and those of the 'to me that looks like . . .' or 'it appears to me . . .' type.

One by one, all the images must be paraded in front of the whole group. At this point, with the input of the group, the director underlines the factors common to different images. If the group is more or less homogeneous, it is likely that many gestures, stances and physical relationships will be similar.

Stage three: the image of the images

The director then proposes that the group form a single image out of all these images – one image which will contain the essential elements of all the others. To help this process, one can start with the image of the principal oppressed, the sculptor. The participants, one by one, must offer their images of the oppressed, using their own bodies. The participants choose the one which is most representative of the group, the most complete one – not the 'best', the 'prettiest', but the most consensual, for whatever reasons (which need not be explained).

Equally, two images can be taken as representative, images that figure two versions, two characteristics, both essential, of the principal oppressed. In this situation two groups of images can then be constructed, if the participants decide that one will not suffice.

Next, around the central image (the image of the oppressed), one by one, other images are constructed, images which have a relationship to the central image and which will complete the tableau, featuring the important elements from the whole collection of individual images. Any significant individual images present in the original parade should be added, but not too many; complexity by all means, but not complication.

Stage four: the dynamisation

To dynamise the image of the images, the director must verify the degree of interrelation of actor and image:

1 Do all the participants *identify* with the images they are presenting, that is, the image that each one is playing? Those who reply in the affirmative stay in these images. The director then asks the other participants if any of them identify with the remaining images, that is, those images incarnated by actors who did not identify with them. If there are affirmative responses, these participants replace the ones who were there first.
2 If, in spite of this, there remain some images with which none of the participants identifies, the director asks them if they *recognise* these images or characters. The process is the same: the actors who recognise their images stay in the image and if there still remain some images or characters unrecognised – this is a rare eventuality – the director asks the same question of the other members of the group.
3 If, in the rarest case, one or more images have still not been recognised, the director asks – as always, first the actors in the image and then the rest – if they feel any *resonance* with these images or characters.

Once these participant/image relationships have been verified, we move on to the three forms of dynamisation:

First dynamisation: interior monologue

For about three minutes (the time allocated will depend on the creativity of the group) all the actors who go to make up the image must utter, without self-interruption, the thoughts their characters are thinking at that particular moment. Without any movement, the actors say everything that comes into their heads, as the characters, not as actors; that is, everything that is related to the situation of the characters they are animating, rather than the theatrical situation which they – as actors – are experiencing. This uninterrupted speech can be extremely difficult. The actors must be warned of this so that the very difficulty will stimulate them. Generally speaking, after a difficult beginning, the actors get used to it and when the three minutes have run out, many may still want to continue. This stage provides great nourishment for the images.

Second dynamisation: dialogue

For a further period of three minutes the actors, still immobile, can engage in dialogue. As they cannot move, if an actor wants to talk to another actor he can't see, or wants to plan an action with him, he has to find a way of doing so in the face of this difficulty – still without movement, using speech alone.

Third dynamisation: desire in action

Very slowly, in slow motion, and this time without uttering a word, without making a sound, the actors move around, trying to show their characters' desires. This form of dynamisation will also last some minutes.

THE PRACTICE

Alzira's threat

In September 1988, in Rio de Janeiro, we applied this technique with a group of around twenty people. We arrived at a collective image in which the principal oppressed was in the centre, seated on the ground – thus unable to walk – hands wedged between his legs – thus ruling out their use for self-defence or attack – eyes riveted to the ground – thus seeing only the ground, and nothing of what was happening around him.

These three elements very often crop up in the images of the principal oppressed: legs that don't walk, hands that cannot grasp anything, eyes that do not see. All the images constructed around this image of the oppressed are images that the oppressed imagines, but cannot actually see. His own image, even without those of the oppressor, is an image of oppression: he is oppressing himself.

Around this central figure, the participants created a veritable wall of statues:

1 someone directly facing the main oppressed, pointing a finger in accusation;
2 someone leaving, or, at least, looking in another direction;

3 two people embracing tenderly, outsiders to the action involving the others;

4 one person standing behind the principal oppressed, hands placed on his head, as if wanting to push him down;

5 another person, further off, in the act of giving him a kick, but not actually making contact;

6 an authoritarian figure, apparently making a speech;

7 a woman, personified by Alzira, in the attitude of someone who wants to go away, with a look of desperation tinged with threat.

These are the images which most affected the group and which cropped up most frequently, in similar forms, in the individual images. The group found figures 1, with pointing finger, and 6, the speech-maker, the most annoying and the most offputting; they represented the most ferocious oppressors. Figures 4 and 5, while apparently the most violent, were perceived as aggressive but not really like oppressors. They had not been internalised by the oppressed, and the fear they engendered was of a purely physical nature. Figures 2 and 3 unsettled people, because in fact they were doing what the oppressed in the group wanted, but lacked the courage, to do; leaving and loving. These two figures represented simultaneously what they desired and what they lacked.

In the end it was with the last image – Alzira, the one who wanted to leave but stayed put, desperate but at the same time threatening – that the majority of the participants identified. They identified more with Alzira than with the principal oppressed, whom they did however recognise as being themselves: 'We are like that: we have legs and yet we don't walk away, we have hands and we hold nothing, we have eyes and we don't see.'

But Alzira moved them most deeply.

We went through the three stages of dynamisation. In the interior monologue, the actor animating the image of the oppressed had considerable difficulty thinking of anything to say except 'no': 'No, I don't want to, I won't go, I can't, I mustn't.' The six images which constituted the wall offered:

1 'I must frighten him, since if he is afraid he will obey me.'

2 Thoughts of the future: another job, another country, friends, a new life.

3 Thoughts of love.

4 'Ah, if only I could really sit on him.'

5 Thoughts of physical violence.

6 Narcissistic self-contemplation.

The seventh image was absolutely coherent in the first two stages of the dynamisation and said no more nor less than one might have expected from her. But she surprised us in the third dynamisation. We will see how later. For the moment, we are dealing with the interior monologues. This image displayed the hatred which fired her against 'those people', her inability to adapt to such mediocre people, her anti-conformity, her need to leave, to flee, no matter where.

The second stage of the dynamisation came out like this.

The images:

1 accused the oppressed of dilettantism, incapability, incompetence, weakness, emptiness;
2 called out to a faraway figure, which we couldn't see, and happily chatted with someone we couldn't hear: they were going away together;
3 spoke of love, as is normal in their situation;
4 was incapable of dialogue, and continued giving voice to his thoughts, along the lines of 'Ah, if only I could . . .'; which struck us as funny, since, with his hands extended to within a few centimetres of the oppressed's neck and being in a position to strangle him, the 'Ah, if only I could . . .' sounded more like an 'Ah, if only I wanted to';
5 revealed his aggressive megalomania: 'This one's first, I'll make an example of him, but afterwards I'll be giving the lot of you a kick up the bum';
6 said things like: 'You don't pay any attention to me, so I am obliged to get tough on you to get you to look at me, to listen to me.'

And Alzira, still following the same line of thought, threatened to leave, said how impossible it was for her to stay, how odious it was for her to be around the others, and so she couldn't stay, she was going, and her departure would make the others suffer, and anything they did to keep her there would be useless, she had definitely decided to leave, that very day, now!

In the third stage of the dynamisation, following the instruction, all the characters showed their desires in action, in movement:

1 pointed his finger, more menacing than ever;
2 went out of the room, left;
3 rolled on the ground;
4 with gestures still suggesting strangulation of the oppressed,

backed off to the wall, as if, in reality, it was he who was being threatened;

5 left at a run, apparently terrified;

6 got onto the table, as if he wanted to take off, to fly, to glide above everything and everyone, far up in the sky, from which vantage point he would be able to see everything and thus be assured, with his own eyes, of his omnipresence.

And Alzira? Well, Alzira made gestures expressive of her threat to leave, revealing her desire to go – but was incapable of taking a single step in any direction, frozen in a physical immobility which was in complete contradiction to her threats.

When the dynamisation was over, I asked Alzira:

'Is your desire then, to stay?'

'No, my desire is neither to stay nor to go. My desire is to threaten. That is my weapon. If I left, I wouldn't be able to threaten any more, since I would be gone. That's why I stay: not because I don't want to leave, but because I desperately want to be able to use this threat. That's what I've discovered. . . .'

Many participants said that they often found themselves in exactly this situation, threatening an action which in reality they did not want to carry out: the abandonment of a companion, of a group. Alzira admitted it:

'At one point in my life, I threatened to commit suicide. I used to tell my husband that one day I would end up committing suicide. At first, this terrorised him. And me too – I suffered a great deal, because everything was mixed up in my head, and, by the very fact of threatening, I ended up believing my own threats, and they terrified me. It came to the point when I used this threat so much that my husband stopped believing me any more; my threats had less and less impact on him, or else perhaps he had resigned himself to becoming a widower. . . . When I realised that the suicide threat was no longer effective, that he was beginning to make fun of it, I had no alternative but to really try and commit suicide. Fortunately the pills weren't strong enough, or there weren't enough of them – the fact is that my attempt failed.'

I disagreed:

'On the contrary, the suicide attempt was a success. If we agree about everything we've said so far, if we are agreed on our understanding of what we have seen today, we must recognise that the suicide attempt was not intended to be suicide: it was an attempt. It came off very well, and, perhaps without your realising it, it was very well done: you chose a pill which was possibly not too strong, you took some of these pills, but possibly not many; it was all just enough to mark it down as a suicide attempt, but not enough to really put your life in danger. And you got what you wanted: your husband started being afraid of your threats again. Am I right?'

'He went into a blue funk.'

The dangerous thing about 'successful attempts' at suicide is their uncertainty. What is the right number of pills? Which pill will be the fatal one? (I think the best approach to attempts of this kind is not to undertake them.)

The suicide attempt and the threat to leave are characteristic of a psychological mechanism which is common enough: a person likes a situation and hates it at the same time; they take pleasure in unhappiness, they revel in their pain. And, it is always difficult for them to abandon the situation which is causing them pain, because it is also a source of pleasure for them. We can enjoy pain, take pleasure in suffering.

So what about the poor image of the principal oppressed? It stayed there, half abandoned. Very little notice was taken of it. But it seemed to us all that it and Alzira were one and the same image, the one in still photo, the other in a film, one immobile, the other in movement, but both staying put. The image of the oppressed depressed us: having hands, why do we not take hold of anything? Having feet, why do we not walk? Having eyes, why is our gaze cast down at the ground? The image of Alzira pained us: why, even when walking, do we always stay on the spot?

The third stage of the dynamisation – when the characters embody their desires in their movements – showed us a surprising thing: the image, as a whole, exploded, each character going off in a different direction. We saw with our own eyes that each image was self-regarding, rejoiced in itself, limited itself to itself. In this synthetic group but also in the original groups, in this *image of the images* but also in the initial images, there was no real structure: all the statues were simply juxtaposed, not engaged in dialogue with each another. It was one large image of many small solitudes.

The women holding Luciano by the legs

At Kassel, in West Germany, in October 1988, a similar thing happened. In the preparatory phase, Luciano constructed an image in which he was at the centre, making vigorous efforts to escape from the clutches of three women who were holding him by the legs. This image dissolved in the image of the images, but, at the end of the process, Luciano asked if we could do the same sequence with his individual image. We agreed. In the *interior monologue*, Luciano spoke of his despair at not being able to get away, since the three women had got him by the legs. In the *dialogue*, Luciano was continually begging them to let go of him. But, in the *desire in action* section, the three women, having to make a great physical effort to hang onto Luciano (an effort they had already complained about in the preceding stages), immediately let go of him and slowly began to leave. Luciano, who had hitherto complained non-stop about his human manacles, his gaolers, did not hesitate: he ran after them, trying to catch them and, strangest of all, to force them to take hold of him:

> 'I wanted to carry on complaining about these women holding me by the legs. When they let go of me I was furious, as I couldn't complain any more. In the monologue and the dialogue, I was saying that I wanted them to let me go, but I didn't actually want them to do what I said. I wasn't looking forward to it at all. In the desire in action phase, I had to do what I actually wanted to do; so I was obliged to try and make them do what I wanted. Do you know what I mean? I have a feeling that, because I couldn't enjoy my pleasure, I at least wanted to be able to revel in my suffering.'

This observation of Luciano's triggered the following reaction from Brigitte:

> 'But what pleasure are you talking about? In most of the individual images we saw people wanting to go without really knowing where, without having anything concrete in front of them. You yourself, Luciano, were trying to run away, but you had the wall in front of you. Where were you running? We've even seen worse, images like my one, arms folded, eyes glued to the ground, sitting on the floor. It's funny how as the image of the group we chose an image of an oppressed person going nowhere; but the bulk of them were like mine: inactive, submissive.'

It was true. Most of the images of the oppressed made by the oppressed themselves are images of resignation. They are not images of defeat in a battle. In Brigitte's case, this was even more evident than she had put it: her hands hid her eyes, but even though they were hidden, her eyes were still downcast, looking at the ground. And her legs were crossed. Why? Why not look, why not see?

> 'I wanted to protect my eyes. . . .'

To protect her eyes, she preferred not to see. And that was a simple statement of fact. We were interpreting nothing. We could state, objectively, that Brigitte could not see. And we were able to show her, in image, the impression her image made on us.

We can use various techniques, with or without speech, immobile or dynamic – in short, we can make theatre out of, and thus speak of, things felt or experienced, without resort to words. Best of all: in deciding of our own free will not to resort to words, in doing Theatre of the Oppressed, we are making theatre, we are making art, since art is an aesthetic language, a language of the senses.

It is true that arms crossed in front of the body can protect it; and also that hands hiding the eyes can protect them. Fists shaken in an attitude of struggle would serve equally well for protection. That we can state categorically. But only Brigitte will know why she chose one and not the other of these forms of protection. We note that she chose this one and not that one. And, perhaps, even knowing full well that legs are for walking, perhaps Brigitte knows why she does not use them.

Brigitte thought for a moment and recapitulated:

> 'We have shown three images of the main oppressed person: mine, on the ground, not seeing anything, not walking, doing nothing with its hands; Luciano's, fleeing or pretending to flee. But there was another one, which also recurred: the body walking in front of one, head turned back, like someone who wants to flee but doesn't want to go away, wants to go elsewhere but without leaving here, someone who wants to go far away while staying close by.'

These were the three principal images. The three had one common characteristic: the oppressed had a relationship with the images which were close by, but no distant objective, as if they could only see the *real image*, not the *ideal image*, as if, in the real image, there was nothing to aim for, no presentation of ideal objectives: 'I don't want that? Then, what do I want? I don't know. . . .' The verb 'to want' fears the complement of a direct object.

Lack of action, going round in circles, the inability to break through an aggressive situation, these are, in general, consequences of the absence of an ideal image. It is that much easier to leave when we know where we want to go. . . . The Spanish poet Antonio Machado wrote: 'Caminante el camino no existe, el camino lo hace el caminante al caminar.' Which can be roughly rendered as, 'The road does not exist, the traveller creates the road by travelling.'

2 The image of the word

This is one of the first techniques I used in image theatre. It consists of choosing a word that is meaningful for the particular group with whom we are working, and asking the participants to make an image of it, using their bodies; the word can be the name of a country, a region, a political party, a profession, a state of mind, a historical character, a recent event; it can be a noun or an adjective; a word which represents something or someone relevant to the group.

The group forms a circle and all the members show their images, simultaneously; then they regroup in families of images which resemble each other. Each family, in turn, vocalises the words inspired by the image.

This technique is described at greater length in my book, *Games for Actors and Non-Actors*.

The images can be constructed with one's own body, with one's own body and someone else's, or with as many bodies and objects as are available.

3 Image and counter-image

This technique is extremely mobilising, since directly or indirectly it involves the whole group. It also has the virtue of preparing the group and its members for new techniques, and for a clearer exposition of the problems they wish to see discussed or analysed.

Stage one: the stories

The director explains the technique and asks which of the participants would like to tell the story of an oppression they have endured and would like to see worked on by the group. The ideal, at this first stage, is that half the participants offer themselves as storytellers. The group thus divides into those who will tell the stories (the protagonists or pilots) and those who will listen (the co-pilots). Each protagonist chooses their co-pilot. The couples distribute themselves around the room. The pilots then quietly recount their stories to their co-pilots. It is important that both protagonist and co-pilot have their eyes closed. If the protagonist keeps her eyes open, she will see the facial reactions of the co-pilot, which might prejudice her telling of the story; her concentration will become more centred on the presence of the co-pilot than on the story that she is telling, and this might prevent her reliving it in depth. It is equally important for the co-pilot to have his eyes closed, so that he will concentrate not on the protagonist but on her story, which he will then be able to experience more fully.

If the co-pilot is not sufficiently sensitised, if his imagination is not sufficiently stimulated, he can – and must – ask questions: 'When? How? Where? What colour? Was it violent? Was it hot? What was the house like? Were there people around? Where were you going? Why did you stop? Why did you not do this or that? What was the idea? Where did it come from? Was he tall? Was he short?' and so on.[●] He can ask whatever questions he likes, while at the same time trying not to cause the pilot to deviate from her main focus: the recollection of whatever details she needs in order to describe and relive the event in question.

The director gives the pilots a reasonable length of time – a quarter of an hour is sufficient in most cases. As not all the couples will take the same length of time, if the director sees that the majority have finished, he should announce this to the remainder, leaving them a few minutes, so as not to interrupt their narratives too brutally. One should be careful to avoid wounding the sensibility of narrator and auditor.

Stage two: the formation of two images

When the stories have been told, the director gathers the participants back together and asks which pairs of pilot (protagonist)

[●] My own experience suggests that questions should be framed in non-judgemental ways, so that the pilot is not forced to 'defend' her action (A.J.).

and co-pilot were able to conjure up clear and strong images of their story. This is why we lay so much stress, in the first stage, on the idea of the co-pilot being a true co-pilot, travelling the same journey as the pilot, not limiting himself to the role of observer, of voyeur; similarly, it is why he must be able to ask questions, because he too must live the scene, feel the same sensations and emotions.

Once the first couple has offered themselves, the second stage begins.

Facing opposite directions, so that they are unable to watch each other, the protagonist and the co-pilot each construct an image of the oppression, with the help of any available objects (anything can be enlisted as vocabulary in this visual language) plus the bodies of as many participants as they need, but trying not to use too many people; it is important that a significant part of the group remain as observers, as witnesses. The protagonist constructs the image of the story she has told, the co-pilot the image of the story he has heard. For neither is this a matter of constructing realistic images which are credible in a literal sense – rather it is about creating real, living, *subjective* images of what has been felt. The intention is not to produce photo-reportage of an event, but its poetic elaboration; truth, not superficiality.

Back to back – without seeing the image that the other one is creating – they construct their images and place themselves in them last, the protagonist in her own position, as herself, the co-pilot in the position of the narrator, the oppressed, as he has understood it.

Stage three: observations on the two images

The director must then direct an exchange of observations around the similarities and differences of the images, with particular reference to the following areas: the position of the protagonist-character (in relation to herself and to others), the distances between characters, the characters present or absent in one or other image, and the number of characters. The two levels of observation should always be characterised as such – the objective, that which is indisputable, since seen by all, and the subjective – remarks that are or could be prefaced by, 'it seems to me'.

It is always interesting to hear what the two builders of the images have to say about what they themselves have done, and their impressions of the other's image.

This stage excites curiosity. Someone always wants to know the original story behind the images. The director must firmly resist this. The only person who needs to know the story as it has been told is the co-pilot. This allows us to work with the *reality of the image*, i.e. the image we see in front of us, and not with the *image of the reality*, which belongs only to the pilot–co-pilot couple. If we know the story, this stage will necessarily be denatured – it will lose its particular analytical power – and the exchange of ideas will become simply a series of guesses, a parlour game.

Stage four: the dynamisations

These can be multiple and various, according to the nature of the images and the group's interest in them.

The three wishes

First, one should use the three wishes mode. The protagonist, availing herself of the magic concession of three wishes, modifies her image three times, with a view to attaining what she really wants. The co-pilot, in his role of protagonist in his own image, can either express what he believes to be the wishes of the protagonist or express his own desires, what he believes the protagonist should wish. Once again, at the end of the three wishes, the director coordinates an exchange of observations on what each partner has done, the course taken by each, the hesi-tations, the decisions, what they did first and what they did last. As before, this should always be done on the two levels: 'this hap-pened in such and such a way, we all saw it' and, 'that seemed to me to mean such and such'. No one interprets, but everyone is allowed to express their projections.

The verification of possible desire and utopian desire

The director asks the participants of the two images to return to their original positions. In slow motion, working in their own images, the protagonist and the co-pilot endeavour to execute the same movements and the same modifications as in the three wishes dynamisation. But this time the other characters in the images, trying their best to sense who they are, what they represent, acting in accordance with that feeling – and making this compatible with what they themselves feel! – acquire a life of their own and, still in slow motion, try either to stand in the way of the protagonist's desires, if they feel they should, or else to support them, if they feel they represent characters who are allies. Once this action is completed, a fresh exchange of ideas and impressions should take place.

The pilots change places

Everyone returns to the original images and the director asks the protagonist and co-pilot to swap places, each taking up exactly the image previously occupied by the other. In these new positions, the two preceding dynamisations are done again. What would the protagonist do if the co-pilot's image was more accurate, contained more truth, than her own?

THE PRACTICE

The dance with the co-pilot

At Kassel, Berta was the first to come forward. She offered to make the image *and* the counter-image. I told her that she had not understood: she must, of course, make the image, because it was she who had told the story, but the making of counter-image fell to the co-pilot. She seemed not to understand a word of this and, in front of the group, continued to ask questions without apparently understanding what she was asking. I use the phrase *in front of the group* advisedly: we were all sitting on the floor and she was standing in front of us. I stood up and asked the co-pilot, Martha, if she was willing to start work. She said yes. I then cut short Berta's questions and asked both to make their images in silence.

Martha immediately constructed her image: two men working (they were painting pictures) and talking, two tables upended on the floor, next to each other, lengthways, forming a high

Berta was very hesitant. She took a long time trying to choose participants for her image, and in the end, looking at us, she said that she didn't need anyone.

wall, and Martha, the co-
pilot, representing Berta
the protagonist, outside,
looking at the wall, unable
to see the two men, who
were also unable to see her.

We discussed the obvious differences: Berta was alone, without
anything or anybody around her to distract our attention. Looking
at her image, we were forced to concentrate on her, since in her
image there was nothing but her, herself, she was alone. In
Martha's image, Martha was trying to see someone who was
unable to see her: two men who were working, chatting, unaware
of her. Berta, we could not be unaware of. Also Berta was not
looking anywhere: she was in front of us as if exhibited. She had
no desire to see anyone, she wanted to be seen by everyone. We
embarked on the three wishes sequence:

These are Martha's wishes, which she executed immediately, without hesitation:

1 She separated the tables, like someone opening a door or knocking down a wall.
2 She angled the two men's faces so that they were looking at her.
3 She kissed the two men and sat down with them on the floor.

With Berta, things went differently. This is her sequence:

1 She made some nervous gestures, uttered a few small sounds of dissatisfaction, but stayed on the spot and remained alone.
2 She took three spectators by the hand, led them on stage, seated them on the ground looking at each other, and stayed alone, outside the triangle, looking around and not finding anything to do.
3 She took the three men and destroyed the triangle by placing them side by side, in such a way as to create two audiences for herself: us and the three men in front of us.

We discussed what we saw: on one side was Martha, kissing the
two men – was this the desire she attributed to Berta or her own

desire? On the other was Berta, performing in front of two audiences.

I decided to continue in my role of generous fairy godmother, and gave them a further three wishes. Both seemed perplexed in the face of this unexpected offer. Martha did nothing more. Berta, still very excited, went on:

> *4th wish*: in a fit of violence, she threw one of the men to the ground, but held back when about to do the same to the others, and spent the rest of the time in a tense, threatening stance;
>
> *5th wish*: she abandoned her aggressive stance and started dancing, all on her own.
>
> *6th wish*: in one rapid movement, she threw the other two men to the ground, invaded the co-pilot's space, destroyed the counter-image, took Martha by the hand and looked her up and down, as if sizing her up, evaluating her . . . and the seconds ticked away and her 6th wish came to a close. . . .

> 'Give me one more!' she demanded, feverishly.

I gave it a moment's thought, which heightened her fever even more.

> 'Give me one more! Go on!'

I allowed her this seventh wish. Berta looked at Martha, who was standing there in a state of paralysis, smiled at her, embraced her, and happily launched into a dance with her, twirling around, frightening the men in the counter-image, knocking into those she had cast to the ground; then, still dancing with her co-pilot, she invaded the wider audience which the rest of us constituted, like a bull in a china-shop, and fell on top of us, completely ignoring us, while we struggled to extricate ourselves from under her.

> 'Did you like it?' she asked, anxiously.

I explained to her that we were not there as spectators of a piece of theatre, to like or dislike a show. We weren't there to see a show. And I told her that the 'dance show' she had offered us was the least important thing as far as we were concerned. What was important was that she had 'offered' us something. She had 'offered' us the dance, the aggression, and the weight of her own body, which was no small thing to offer! She had offered us something we had not asked for. She had imposed her offers on us. She had not wanted to know what we wanted: she was giving us what she wanted to give us. She was thrusting her gifts down our throats, and making us swallow them. She was ignoring our wishes, just as, in her image, she had ignored our presence, showing herself on her own, after having looked at and evaluated us.

Berta had shown her lack of interest in those she wished to interest in herself – like a cinema star, loving her audience but not the people it is made up of. As for us, we were protecting ourselves from this aggression like the two men in the counter-image, raising barricades: they with their barricades of tables, we with our barricades of words.

In Berta's first image, other people were so far away that she did not see them, did not place them on stage. But at that moment, we were the other people, we who were close by and unseen by her. She would not see us, but she wanted us to see her.

This wanting to be seen by those she did not want to see was revealed aesthetically in the counter-image: Martha the co-pilot wanted to enter, but without being able to see the men who were within. But in the three wishes dynamisation, it is clear that Martha was showing her own wishes, her own desire to be with others, and not Berta's desire.

The people used in the counter-image and in Berta's last wishes were all men. The women in the group were completely ignored. Berta had made her audience out of men, had invaded the group of men in the counter-image, had recognised herself in Martha, had loved herself in loving her, and, enfolding her in her arms, had thrown herself onto the men in the audience.

Though she loved herself and saw herself surrounded by men, she still directed her aggression towards these men. First she wanted them to see her enjoying her solitary dance; then, she physically chastised them. She was annoyed by their passivity, which, though one of the rules of the game, part of our technique, struck her as indifference.

Her relationship with Martha had been difficult and ambiguous. She had looked at her in amazement, had evaluated herself in evaluating her, contemplated herself in contemplating her, recognised herself in recognising her, accepted herself in accepting her. She had enjoyed the solitary dance with her, the dance with herself. And, dancing with herself, she had fallen heavily onto a number of inert men.

The dance was a source of pleasure, especially the dance *à deux*, her with herself. The inertia was a source of pain.

Lord Byron: a time for leaving

In one of his many fine poems, Lord Byron says: 'There is a time for departure, even when there is no certain place to go.' This is true: many a time we feel an urgent and unsettling need to leave, to go away. Where to? We don't know. We only know that we have to go. But without knowing where to go, leaving becomes extremely difficult.

In Graz, in October 1988, Paulo had an image he wanted to make: there was a woman, behind a table, trying to catch him. The participants insisted on calling this woman 'the mother', which did not rule out the possibility that she might have been 'the wife' or 'the sister'. Whether actually a mother or not, she was truly the incarnation of 'the mother' in this image.

The image comprised only these three elements: a table in the middle, which acted as an obstacle and a means of separation, but also as an object unifying the bodies of Paulo and his 'mother' in a single image. Hermann, the co-pilot, sculpted the same image.

I asked both of them to try *zooming out*: as in a film, the camera backs away, and by enlarging the field of vision, allows sight of other characters, other scenery.

Without overmuch reflection, Hermann put three characters in front of the image of the protagonist, Paulo (played by Hermann): two girls and a boy, modelled as if running.	After a great deal of thought, Paulo added no-one to his image. He merely changed the direction of his gaze: instead of looking at the wall of the room, which was far away, he now looked at the window, which was slightly closer.

We used the three wishes mode:

Hermann immediately forgot about 'the mother' and joined the three people.	Paulo looked back and fixed the mother with a steely gaze.
Hermann hugged the two girls, excluding the boy.	Paulo gazed at the window.
Hermann abandoned the girls and moved forwards.	Paulo went to the window and looked out.

Hermann chose the door by the entrance, full of people. Paulo chose the window, which looked out onto empty space.

Paulo wanted to get away from where he was. He examined the place, he had a relationship with the person he wanted to abandon, he looked at her, felt her presence, looked at her again, sized up his space, was conscious of himself in that space, and when he looked outside was gazing at the infinite, the void, where there was nothing, where there was nobody.

Hermann, rather than simply go, wanted to go somewhere. First he joined the group, then he removed the women, and after that he proceeded on his journey to a place where people were to be found. The one wanted to get away from where he was, the other wanted to go to where he was not. The point of reference of the former was precisely the thing he wished to abandon and which, in serving as his point of reference, fascinated and imprisoned him. The latter, projecting his desire further, using his energies not to separate himself from something close by but to reach something far off, succeeded, dynamically, in moving forwards, while the former succeeded only in looking backwards.

There is a time for leaving.

4 The kaleidoscopic image

This technique seeks to exploit the imprecisions, ambiguities, ambivalences and polysemies, which may be mingled with the perception of a scene or an event. Sometimes we need to know the precise limits of a scene, assure ourselves of its 'uniqueness', its 'univocity'. At other times it is not exact lines of demarcation that we must seek, but superpositions, double meanings, the nebulous, the fields of 'could be yes, could be no', 'maybe', 'who knows?', because it is precisely there, in the realm of supposition, in the indeterminate, in the hidden, that something is concealed, some piece of knowledge which can be aesthetically revealed, seen, sensed, felt. I reiterate that whatever therapeutic effect the Theatre of the Oppressed may have, this effect is obtained through aesthetic means alone, via the senses, because art is the medium we are dealing with.

This technique deals, therefore, with the incidental and the aleatory, which can be determinants.

It works with raw material, with wheat and chaff, with gold ore, with uncut marble, from which the features of the statue appear.

Here, it is not a matter of deciding that this is this and not that; this is this and that, and something else as well. Here, the task is not to ask why; here, things are as they are, quite simply because they are as they are – but they might also be different.

Stage one: the improvisation

The protagonist 'writes' and 'directs' her story, in which she will play herself. She chooses the other actors, who will faithfully follow her instructions and, within the limits imposed upon them, will also themselves create, imagine, experiment: an improvisation is always a combination of what has been told to the actor who is improvising, and her own experience of her own life.

Stage two: the formation of images

Using their own bodies, the participants show images of the perceptions, feelings, emotions, aroused in them by the scene and the characters. They create two categories of image: those relating to the protagonist, and those relating to the antagonist or antagonists. Preferably, the scene should be centred on a dialogue: the protagonist and another. This formation of images should be executed with resort to the third category of relation to images, resonance, not solely on the basis of identification or recognition.

To reiterate: there is identification when the participant thinks, feels and says, 'He is like me, I am thus'; there is recognition when he thinks, feels and says, 'This person is not me, but I know who he is, I know people like him.' In the first case, as the protagonist (or an image of the protagonist), he will be playing himself on stage, reliving his own emotions. In the second case, he will be 'interpreting', that is, living the part of himself which is brought into play.

With resonance, a much greater degree of imprecision operates. Here, the participant is saying, 'This reminds me of such and such a person, such and such an event, situation, feeling; to me, this seems like that.' Or equally, 'That could have been different, he should have acted in this manner; if he had done something else, everything would have turned out differently.' Resonance can, of course, include identification and recognition.

The images created in response to the initial improvisation are frozen statues.

Stage three: the constitution of couples and their witnesses

Each image seeks, in subjective fashion, its own complement. Either the two actors who make up the couple find each other spontaneously, or else, if two actors both choose the same third person as their complement, it is up to the third to choose which he will form a couple with. At least five couples must be constituted for a good kaleidoscope to be possible.

Each couple will then be attended by a witness. This witness has a dual function: to reinforce the aesthetic space and to furnish testimony. She reinforces the aesthetic space because in her presence the two actors will be conscious of being seen. They will live the scene on stage and, at the same time, they will be showing it to a witness.

Stage four: the fair

In this fourth stage, within the same room, the couples thus constituted improvise their scenes simultaneously, each in front of their witness. This multiplicity also has a dual function: it liberates the actors from the excessive pressure of an audience, allowing them to be in a privileged space; they are in solitary intimacy – each of the other participants only concerning themselves with their own scene – but they are also observed by their witness, who shares in their solitary intimacy.

Before starting the improvisation, using their images as the starting point, each couple decides (1) where it is going to happen; (2) who each of them is; (3) what they want from each other.

The protagonist and antagonist from the original scene are allowed to wander around this 'fair'. The director and another participant, neither actor nor witness, can also observe the couples improvising simultaneously. But they must above all *observe the protagonist observing the couples*: her movements from one scene to the next, the time she spends watching each scene, all her bodily movements, which are, in themselves, a 'discourse', a 'writing', and which can, afterwards, be 'read', so that the protagonist can recognise what she has done and the manner in which she did it.

This 'fair' almost inevitably turns into a brouhaha. To avoid too much confusion, after a few minutes of free improvisation by the couples, the director asks them to continue in the *softly softly* mode. The actors, already stimulated, already 'charged', intensified by the first part of the improvisation, will tend, by the use of this mode, further to deepen their perceptions, feelings and emotions.

Stage five: the reimprovisations

After the 'fair', we move on to reimprovisations. Each couple presents itself in front of the whole group, and their witness reports back on all she has seen and all she has felt and noticed. The actors cannot speak before the reimprovisation. After this testimony, the couple reimprovise the scene, trying this time to *show*, more intensely, what they had improvised before, with the goal either of corroborating the witness's testimony or of denying it and, by means of this magnified improvisation, presenting a contradictory testimony.

And so, one after the other, preceded by their witnesses, each couple must pass in front of the group. At the end of each reimprovisation, everyone, including the actors, can talk about their perceptions and sensations. They can reveal their *admiration*⊚ for what they have seen, thus allowing the group to *admire their own admiration*, to be astonished at their astonishment, to wonder at their wonder.

Stage six: the discussion

The director then opens a discussion on the totality of the experience. The discussions that took place directly after the reimprovisations will have centred mainly on the things everyone had just seen, and may not have been related back to the whole ensemble of improvisations.

⊚ From the Latin *admiratio*: the action of wondering or marvelling in front of something extraordinary or unexpected. The important point of this emphasis on admiration is to rekindle a sense of surprise and to question the common, unspoken assumption that a group of individuals is surprised by the same things, and conversely, takes the same things for granted. To take things for granted is to accept them; to be surprised by them is to challenge them (A.J.).

THE PRACTICE

The captain in the mirror

In April 1989 I was working in Berne, in Switzerland, with a group of therapists, educationalists and others. I presented this technique. A long silence ensued before anyone came forward. Finally, Dominique offered himself:

'I have a story to tell, but I would need a mirror, a big mirror, and there isn't one here.'

I told him that we could always use the wall as a mirror, but my suggestion appeared not to satisfy him. Someone remembered that one of the curtains in the room hid just such a mirror, a huge one. We rushed to the curtain and the mirror was there, a fine old mirror, imposing in its gilt frame. I should explain that we were working in the hall of a beautiful, very ancient, medieval château. . . .

Dominique looked at the mirror.

'Yes . . . the one I'm thinking of was pretty much like that. . . . Maybe even a little larger. . . . '

I asked him if he wanted to improvise in front of the real mirror or if he would prefer to use the wall as a mirror. He preferred the wall, and I was glad he decided in favour of it: onto this opaque wall it would be easier for him to project his memories and relive his emotions. I asked him to choose the actor who would represent his antagonist, and he chose a small, thin man, to whom he gave his instructions. The improvisation began.

It was a violent scene. Like all Swiss people, Dominique had to do a certain number of days a year of military training, up until the age of fifty. The Swiss army numbers very few professional soldiers and officers in its ranks. Dominique told how one day he had been called into the captain's office to be disciplined over a minor offence. The captain ordered him to look in the mirror, and, in the mirror, to look at the two of them, Dominique and the captain. And to give him a military salute, still looking in the mirror.

'What do you see there?'

'I see myself.'

'No! You do not see yourself, you see a soldier! Look carefully, here you are not yourself! Here, you are a soldier! A soldier in the Swiss army! And what else do you see?'

'I see you.'

'No! You do not see me, you see a captain. Look at the stripes: that man there is a captain in the Swiss army!'

'Yes, *mon capitaine. . . .*'

'I don't know what you do outside here, what profession you are engaged in, that does not interest me at all! All I know is that in here you are a mere private. Have you got that, soldier? Here you are an insignificant soldier, a nobody, and I am your captain, a captain in the Swiss army! Is that understood, little Private Nobody?'

'Yes, captain.'

The scene went like this: Dominique reduced to his condition of Private Nobody, and the captain exalted in his guise of dashing professional captain in the Swiss army. In reality, this scene was played out quite a number of times, the captain in question trying on each occasion to assert his superiority more strongly.

We passed on to the resonances stage.

The scene had 'resonated' intensely with all the participants. Almost all wanted to show how they had experienced Dominique's scene with the captain. People got into couples, witnesses offered themselves, we did the 'fair', listened to the witnesses, the scenes were reimprovised. Three improvisations were chosen, those most representative of the intense and morbid relationship between the captain and Dominique:

1 The captain imposing on Dominique a relationship which was sexual in its symbolism. He paraded himself in front of him, resplendent in uniform and stripes, as a sexual object. He showed all his virtues in opposition to the soldier's inferiorities, like a sort of Miss Julie◎ making love to her valet, and at the same time humiliating him, like the daughter in *Mr Puntila and His Man Matti.*◎ The captain paraded like a peacock fanning its tail. The task of punishing Dominique was of little consequence to him; what he really wanted was to be admired, exalted, and he needed the soldier's presence so that he himself could believe in his pretended beauty. The actor playing the captain even executed a few dance steps, performing a little ballet in which he himself was the ballerina.

2 The captain inflicting himself on Dominique in a sadistic relationship. At every opportunity, he would repeat the most wounding epithets: 'inferior', 'good for nothing', and even 'soldier'. . . . At the same time he would rehearse Dominique's vulnerability: 'Outside you may be whoever you like; in here

◎ From August Strindberg's play *Miss Julie* (1888).

◎ *Mr Puntilla and His Man Matti*, an early Brecht play.

you are nothing, and you are obliged by law to come here every year. And since you are obliged to come here every year, and since you are nothing here, it stands to reason that outside you are also nothing.' The scene mutated almost into physical torture; the actor gave out the sorts of signal which are the forerunners of actual bodily harm.

3 The captain in mid-identity crisis and needing Dominique to affirm his own identity as captain. He needed an inferior being to attest that he was indeed the captain, he needed to 'see' himself in that reflection, to verify this captain/soldier relationship, in which he was not soldier but captain. He behaved like an actor dressing in his character's costume and looking at himself in a mirror the better to play his part, the better to feel it.

Other resonances were shown, some from the captain's perspective, others from Dominique's, but the above three touched me most, particularly the last.

Why the last?

Switzerland is the only country in the world condemned to live in peace. The currencies of the whole world circulate in Switzerland, and it is in no country's interest for Switzerland to go to war, since it would have to abandon its banking neutrality. During the Second World War, armies killed each other and murdered the inhabitants of the planet by the million. Neutrality spared the Swiss the horrors of war, the massacres, the systematic slaughter, the methodical destruction. The rivers of blood steered clear of immaculate Switzerland and its full, sealed coffers.

And yet the Swiss needed, and still need, to believe that they inhabit a country and not a banking zone – a kind of giant Wall Street; to see themselves as a country, they need to look like other countries. All countries have an army. So Switzerland has to have an army, even though it is useless. What's the use of an army which doesn't go to war? Why plan battles which will never be fought? Why bother drawing up tactics and strategies which will end up in the dustbin?

It is for this reason, I think, all things considered, that it is understandable that Swiss captains should not believe in the career of officer, just as I can understand how the admirals of the Paraguayan or Bolivian navy might not think of themselves as real sailors. If you never go to sea, you're not a sailor; if you don't make war, you're not a soldier; people who don't make love cannot think of themselves as lovers.

Strange as it may seem, we all worked on the scene thinking primarily of the captain, which did not however bother Dominique, who told us that he had learnt a lot from this work. Reflecting on the scene, we asked ourselves whether the captain was a psychotic, incapable of assuming his identity or, by contrast, whether he was a lucid man who – even if only on a sensory level – was capable of being a non-captain, a sailor on dry land. Having a real gun in his hand did not make him a real soldier. If all the real weapons belonging to the Swiss army could have been magically transformed into toys, it would have made no difference to the recent history of Switzerland. And that is not a judgement, it is a fact.

Switzerland is a such a small country, and so full of contrasts. . . . As well as playing host to four official languages, each canton has its own legislation which sometimes contradicts principles which we would consider to be national matters. For example, in at least one canton women do not have the right to vote.⑩ In this canton, each elector must turn up at the vote with his sword. And as the women don't have swords. . . .

Order is necessary, in Switzerland more so than in any other country. Disorder is permissible, as long as it is well ordered. The carnival in Basle starts at exactly five o'clock in the morning and finishes precisely at midday, on designated days of the week. Not a few minutes after midday; midday on the dot. After midday, it is forbidden.

As in most countries, drugs are forbidden. But at any hour of day or night the passer-by can witness a terrible spectacle which takes place every day in the Platzspitz in Zurich. A central location, beside the main railway station, the Hauptbahnhof and next to an important museum, this is not far from the river Limmat. In this square, every day tens, sometimes hundreds, of young or not so young drug addicts gather. They hang around there chatting, observed by the civil police who patrol and, with varying degrees of discretion, identify the new addicts. A state bus is parked there, where the addicts can exchange used syringes for new ones – the state trying, by this means, to limit the rapid growth of AIDS cases; if they want, the addicts can also meet a duty social worker there to talk or plan a treatment with her. In the most central point of this park, various little stands lend the aspect of a street market to a place where dealers sell all sorts of drugs available on the market, at market prices.

⑩ This is the 'demi-canton' Appenzell-Rhodes Extérieures, one of whose citizens even declared in all sincerity: 'At my place, it is the wife who gives the orders. And, as she is against the vote for women, at the next referendum to decide whether or not women should have the right to vote, in obedience to my wife, I shall vote against the vote for women.' (La Suisse, 24 April 1989). In spite of that, women won, and now they can vote even in the Appenzell-Rhodes Extérieures (A.B.).

I was working in a youth culture centre and to get there I used to cross the park every day. One day I saw two young lovers there, tenderness incarnate: the boy's arm fondly around the girl, she with a syringe stuck into her arm. When she had finished injecting the drug, she started opening and closing her hand, to produce a faster circulation of the drug in her bloodstream, a more immediate and stronger effect. Hypnotised, I watched the two of them gazing at each other tenderly, not seeing me; they were on a trip. They were travelling far from Zurich, far from Switzerland where drugs are forbidden, except – perhaps – if the drug addicts behave themselves, create no scandal and confine themselves to this park. Just like Speakers' Corner in London, where the citizen can say whatever she wants, where she can even swear to have seen the Pope kissing the queen of England, since the police will be on hand to guarantee her right to free speech (as long as she stays at Speakers' Corner). . . .

Let us return to our scene. By acting in this way, by forcing the young soldier to look at his image – by obliging him to see the superficiality of things, to look at his uniform while he spoke – the captain succeeded in penetrating and devastating the most intimate areas of this young man's unconscious: he forced him to regress to his earliest sensations and infantile emotions, to his primal fears and certainties.

In fact, the mirror plays an essential role in the formation of the identity of the child, for whom all is fluid, all is uncertain, all is terrifying. Everything places him in front of the unknown; even repetitive facts, events which happen every day at the same times, are experienced by the child – in a catastrophic manner – for the first and last time, for the only time. If the sun goes down, for the child eternal night has fallen; if mother isn't there, she is dead for ever; hunger is the premonition of death. The child does not know that everything repeats itself or can repeat itself. He does not know what we can command, nor what commands us. For him, everything happens as a torrent of phenomena obeying no laws; the child has not acquired the codes of the adult.

None the less, in front of the mirror, the child discovers his first identity, his first power, his first voluntary repetition – he learns that he can make things repeat themselves. He sees himself, his image in the mirror, constant. He makes a gesture, the image repeats it. He smiles and sees his smile. 'I am he and he is me, but it is I who give the orders. I raise my hand, and my image raises his, I laugh, he laughs. I close my eyes and the image disappears. I am he, but it is I who give the orders, it is I who am the boss, the captain. I am the captain of my image, which obeys me.'

In penetrating the mirror, the child learns to command, to be the subject: he commands his image in the mirror. From this to theatre is only one short step: instead of seeing himself in the mirror, he looks at himself 'on stage' and sees himself directly. But the mirror is his first stage.

The terrible cruelty of this captain resided in the act of penetrating this image himself as well, himself crossing the frontier of the mirror – the soldier's unconscious – and, inside, in the reflected image and in Dominique's unconscious, taking from him the only power that we all possess: the power to be. Forced to look at himself in the mirror – his primary and principal conquest as a human being endowed with imagination – Dominique renounced that power, he ceased to be. He became a new being, the being demanded by the captain; he was no longer the person he wanted to be. In performing a military salute, he saw himself deprived of the power to command his own image. The mirror is an intimate, personal object. The captain violated Dominique's intimacy.

This apparently innocuous punishment in reality contains at least one of the essential objects of other more common tortures: i.e. annihilating the individuality, the identity of the victim of torture. When torturers force their victims to undress, the thought of sparing clothes from the imminent flow of blood is far from their minds; they really want the person to undress (French: *déshabiller*). Words sometimes serve as a means of concealment for the thinking behind them, but they can also reveal that thinking. In this case, the word reveals. *Déshabiller* literally means to undo oneself of habits, of those habits which cover us, habits we have chosen, a result of our freedom of choice, a part of us. It is this part of us that the torturers wish to eliminate, so that we lose our chosen identity, the identity visible in our habits, and regress to our animal identity, the corporeal, physical, sensitive identity which is subject to pain and suffering, which is vulnerable.

The victim of torture is obliged to divest herself of all that individualises her, to strip away her history, and, from the historic individual she was, carrying with her her defeats and victories, a profession and a family, neighbours and friends, she now becomes a mere human body: a head, trunk and limbs, sensitive and vulnerable. Other elements obviously come into this torturer–tortured relationship, elements of a sexual order: the naked body is the source of both ultimate pleasure and ultimate pain.

It was with this goal of using torture to destroy the victim's identity that, during the recent periods of dictatorship in many Latin American countries, torturers would rape wives in front of their husbands. They hoped to destroy the identity called 'husband', 'man', 'companion', the identity of the person designated by society as 'the protector', 'the head of the family', 'the spouse'. It was with this goal in mind that they would torture the son in front of the father. Or, even more horrific and more tragic, they would force one member of a family to torture another.

'What you are on the outside doesn't interest me; here, you are just a soldier,' said the captain.

And this person who wanted to be an engineer – who knew how to be an engineer – lost his title. This person who had a name became a number, any old number, arbitrary, worth as much – or as little – as any other.

Since what he was 'on the outside' did not matter, since 'in here' he would always be a soldier, and 'on the outside' he would always be obliged to come 'in here' once a year, what he was 'in here' became his true identity and what he was 'on the outside' a semblance, a trick, a mere theatrical presentation. The truth became the mirror instead of the person the mirror reflected.

In front of the mirror, the captain gives the order: 'You are not yourself! You are the soldier we see in the mirror. You are him, but it is he who commands you and he is under my command!'; all the opposite of what Dominique, as a baby, had learnt by himself. The meeting of army and childhood begets such contradictions.

All these thoughts came to us by means of this theatrical, aesthetic dynamisation of diverse images, fruits of the resonances provoked in the participants by the initial improvisation. These resonances were shown to us aesthetically, and not merely verbally. What Dominique discovered and learnt – and what we all learnt with him – was given to him by means of theatre; by means of images, sounds, colours, distances, words, rhythms, melodies and movements.

'It was as if the barracks suddenly came back, like in a dream,' said Dominique. 'But this time, you were with me, and I was awake. So I was able to enter my dream as if I was entering the mirror and the dream no longer frightened me. Here, it is I who give the orders, so I can understand things better.'

We learnt something that day, we and Dominique, and that something changed us. For the better.

The strangled word

In Rio de Janeiro, in May 1989, Hermano proposed a scene featuring him and his son. The two of them are talking on the telephone; Hermano cannot go and pick up his son because, that very day, he has a theatre session with me; he tries to arrange another date for their meeting. They talk and talk, invisible to each other, each at one end of the phone. And when I say talk, I really mean talk . . . they knew how to talk.

We went through the process. Some fairly obvious images were shown, along with other more penetrating ones, until the very last one, which made a great impression on us. The actor portraying the image of the son was completely bent double. His head was almost touching the floor. His back was turned on the actor playing his father; the latter, seated on a chair, was staring fixedly into empty space. The father talked and talked and talked, while his body remained completely immobile. With him, everything came out in speech. The son began to respond with strangled words. For instance, he would be saying 'no', but each 'no', although still the same word, would come out as a different word. At one moment it would be a 'noooooooooooooooo', poignant as a scream, then 'nonononononononononononono!', like the rattle of a machine-gun, then 'no . . . o . . o . . o . . o . . o . . o', like the echo of a body falling into a chasm.

The word 'no' was strangled, stabbed, murdered with a bloody fury. The signifier (the word) left its signified (the original meaning) far behind, became an onomatopoeic cry, changing its meaning on each utterance. The word became an object.

Hermano reflected:

> 'The trouble is that we talk on the telephone, without seeing each other. And with this kind of conversation between father and son, it should be face to face, eye to eye.'

As everything was being conveyed by speech, speech pronounced at a distance, this speech in reality served more to conceal than to reveal. Why had the father and mother separated? Why had this separation affected the son in this way, why had it been such a blow that he felt abandoned? Why did the father want to meet him at the assigned hour to converse, if not to mark the boundaries of their common life? And what was the father like outside these boundaries? The son's anxiety, his desire to meet up with his father again, his unconscious guilt – speech hid all this, restricting itself to the fixing of a timetable: 'This evening, tomorrow morning, Sunday afternoon I will be free, maybe between two and four, or from nine to midday, or now, or later, or maybe, who knows, maybe never again.'

Words reveal but they also conceal. In the present case, they concealed. That is why the actor-son felt the need to lacerate them. And by this process the father, Hermano, was able to sense, *aesthetically*, that in his encounters with his son he used speech in place of speaking, that is, he used words to hide, to evade questions. He talked about the weather, classes, work, elections, but he was not listening to nor answering his son's unverbalised, but none the less intense, question:

'What about me?'

That was all the son wanted to know: 'What about me?' And it was also the very thing the father was stopping himself discovering, using words as his cover. The son then murdered every one of these words, opening a wound in the father, a hurt equal to his own. This murder made their mutual understanding aesthetically possible, the son exploding syntax, pronouncing disconnected, mutilated words, words in tatters.

It'll come. . . .

In Berne, Mathilde proposed a scene in which her husband was refusing to contribute financially to the upbringing of their daughter, but demanding the right to see her when he pleased. During the *resonances* stage, the participants are entitled to show images of anything that 'resonates' for them, which is why we call this technique *kaleidoscopic*. They can show for example:

1 what they would have done in the protagonist's place;
2 what they would have liked the protagonist to have done;
3 those actions the protagonist did do which weakened her;
4 images of the antagonist, of his power, of his weapons;
5 memories, even vague ones, of themselves in similar situations.

Thanks to this panoply of possible responses, two young women showed two images of a strong, forceful Mathilde, refusing to accord her husband any rights unless he also accepted his duties. These images were the result of a tiny, hidden element, as yet weak, but none the less present in Mathilde's behaviour, a part of her self which had not yet reached the stage of powerful self-expression.

One of the hypotheses of the Theatre of the Oppressed is that knowledge acquired aesthetically is already, in itself, the beginning of a transformation. The improvisations over, I asked the two young girls if they believed that Mathilde was 'like that', the way they had shown her. They said yes, she was. I put the question to Mathilde. She answered:

'Not yet, but it'll come. . . . '

5 The images of the image

This technique should not be confused with *The image of the images*, in which we try to create a single, synthetic image of all the images sculpted by the participants. Here, it works the other way round: the participants must sculpt various images starting from a single original image.

Stage one: the improvisation

A normal improvisation, in which the protagonist explains to the participants how they should improvise, giving each person their motivation (their will, their desire) and their characterisation (how this desire disports itself, what form it takes, what characteristics it has).

Stage two: the formation of images

After the improvisation, one by one, anything between three and five participants each sculpt an image of the scene as they perceived it, using the same actors as took part in the original improvisation. When the first participant has finished sculpting his image, the actors improvise the same scene again, but now in the image as it has been re-sculpted; each actor can make any movements he wants, as long as they don't fundamentally alter his own image or the relationships between his image and the

⑩ There is a tremendous temptation, when working in this or any other of the techniques that use fixed images, for the participants to break out of their image in order to perform a particular action which their bodily stance renders especially difficult; inasmuch as it is possible, this temptation should be resisted. Often it is as a result of this very constraint, inbuilt into the image and thrown into sharp relief when it tries to do something for which it appears physically ill designed, that the most revealing (and sometimes hilarious) insights about the nature of the image come to the fore. For example, in a recent workshop we saw an image of a man involved in an argument with his partner over rights of access to their child; the image was a macho stance with legs apart and arms firmly crossed – when it came to changing the child's nappies, the man found the operation a near impossibility. However, as with all rules in the Theatre of the Oppressed, this rule can be broken, and usually when it is broken it signifies a change in the dynamic; the character breaks out of the image because he simply cannot bear it any more, it is no longer applicable or useful (A.J.).

others.⑩ The general structure of the scene must stay unchanged. The same process is then carried out, in the same way, with the second participant, who sculpts her image, on which a further improvisation will be done, and so on till the last.

We will thus have reimprovised the same original improvisation several times according to the images constructed by the participants. Obviously each reimprovisation will show the same scene in a new light, from a new angle. The same words, the same phrases, acquire new meanings, sometimes barely nuanced, sometimes even completely opposed to the sense in the original improvisation. The same meanings do not, however, remain attached to the same words each time, as the mediating image is different and the image 'filters' the words, lending them its own colour.

THE PRACTICE

From July to August 1989, in Rio de Janeiro, I directed a workshop with pupils and teachers from New York University. Mary suggested a scene: her boyfriend was due in court on a drug-taking charge which, according to her, was false. Mary was ready to appear as a witness for the defence. Her parents, worried by this, had asked to see her to discuss the matter with her. She met up with her father, her mother and her brother.

First improvisation: the father discovers that Mary has been cohabiting with her boyfriend for more than a year. He is flabbergasted to learn that his daughter is no longer an innocent virgin, but a woman (these things happen, alas, even in the United States . . .). The son immediately weighs in, in support of his father. Mary asks her brother if he has yet lived with a woman. The brother answers that he has, yes, but that he would never marry either this woman or any other woman who would agree to live with him before marriage. Mary seeks the support of her mother who, like a stereotypical mother, thinks only of serving the tea and biscuits, appealing for calm, changing the subject, talking about the weather and the neighbours, asking them to keep their voices down . . . and paradoxically succeeds only in making everyone else even more annoyed.

Further improvisations: the images which were made afterwards showed the mother shared between the other three; the father and the son, two men united against Mary; the son hanging on to his father's coat-tails; the father looking outside, wanting to leave and obliged to stay; and above all, Mary's immense hostility towards her brother. Mary could abandon mother and father, she could hide her life from them, she could even ignore them. But when it came to her brother, it was a completely different matter. She could not forgive him. He was her age, part of the same scene, he hung around with friends who thought like her and he was turning into a traitor. Mary could not forgive him his fear of their father, which was making him side with ideas he did not believe in.

I then proposed a fresh improvisation: Mary alone with her father. And, curious as it may seem, things went less badly. The father, though he wanted to, never got to the point of turning the encounter into a police interrogation. It was as if, in front of the family, he felt obliged to be the stern father. Alone with his daughter, he no longer behaved like the head of the family, but like a father, and the conversation flowed calmly, without sudden emotional outbursts. There was time to exchange ideas, to gain some mutual understanding.

In the first improvisation, Mary had wanted to analyse the hostility of her relationship with her father; in the last, her exclusive antagonism towards her brother became evident: there lay her real conflict. It was as if the whole familial structure, with father, mother and brother all present at the same time, had aggressive tendencies towards Mary which were not present in each individual member of the family in isolation. The family was more than the sum of its parts.

6 The projected image

I have described this old technique in detail in *Games for Actors and Non-Actors*.[◎] It consists of constructing a dynamic image and asking the participants to do a forum on it, in which each person projects their own feelings onto the scene, 'interpreting' it in their own way, and, still in the dynamic image but in silence, trying solutions and alternatives.

Originally, we used this technique with a synthetic image as its starting point. Lately, I have begun to use it starting from any image a participant has constructed to tell her story, through the image and without words. Since images are polysemic, one always learns something from the experience of others. While I want to

◎ Due to a translator's error (this translator) in some early editions of *Games for Actors and Non-Actors* this technique is erroneously referred to as The Screen Image, which is in fact a different technique described later in this book (A.J.).

signify my experience by means of my image (the signifier), other participants will project on to this same signifier other possible signifieds.

7 The image of the hour

This prospective technique is very simple and very useful for the rapid mobilisation of a group and the aesthetic verification of its common elements.

Stage one: the game

The director asks the group to walk round the room. From time to time she gives three sorts of instructions: (1) *time*; (2) *image*; (3) *action*. The *time* command is a successive sequence of key times of day or night. On some occasions this time is specified exactly: midday, two o'clock, four o'clock, ten o'clock, midnight, three in the morning, eight in the morning, ten in the morning. At other times, it is vaguer: the end of the afternoon, evening, early in the morning, at night, etc. At yet other times, when the director feels it important, she can specify even the day of the week: Saturday night, Sunday afternoon. Or even call to mind special dates: six in the afternoon on election day, first thing in the morning on your birthday, quarter to midnight on New Year's Eve. Or even unique dates: the day of the death of a president in office. . . .

So, the director announces the time and the participants prepare themselves. Then she gives the command 'image!' and all the participants simultaneously adopt the image of what they habitually do, ritualistically (or exceptionally in the unique cases) at that time and on that day. Finally the director will say 'action!' and the participants engage in dialogue with the (imagined) characters to whom they are normally relating at that time and on that day. Each actor remains immersed in, limited to, his personal world, without contact with the rest of the actors.

At the command 'Stop!', all stop and prepare for the next stage.

Stage two: the discussion

The director centres the discussion on what happened for each of the participants, and the points of contact, of similitude, between what they did or experienced: at what point did each or all feel at the peak of their powers? At what point did the energy lapse? Which were the most agitated moments? When did they feel most mobile? Most at ease? What relationships did they have with other people? With animals? With the telephone? With the television set? At what moments are the actions they carry out motivated by desire and at what moments do they do things because they are forced to by signals or by obligations? At which moments do they feel constrained, at which others are they happy? At what moment did each person feel the same as everyone else? At what moment did they feel unique?

8 The ritual gesture[©]

One actor makes a movement that reproduces some aspect of a ritual of her everyday life, then she stops at a crucial point. The others, recognising it, enter on stage and complete the scene she is playing, with their bodies. No words are used. After a number of participants have joined in, the director can enquire where each person thought they were, what they thought they were doing. With a very homogeneous group, there will often be a large degree of 'accurate' recognition, as these will probably be shared rituals. With less homogeneous groups there may be a wide variance – one person thought she was at work in the office, another thought she was in school; as always with this work, the contradictory assumptions are at least as interesting as the complementary assumptions.

[©] This technique is discussed in more detail in *Games for Actors and Non-Actors*.

SOCIAL CODE, RITUAL AND RITE

To walk on the right or left is a social code; a ritual is a sequence of movements, dialogues, actions that we perform when our hearts are no longer in them. Rituals mechanise us; for the most part, they are unconscious and not easily seen. A rite is a conscious spectacle designed to be seen, such as the investiture of a president, or a formal wedding.

Stage one: the model

The model is the scene or play, image or sequence of images, or dynamic image, that we work on, theatrically; the starting point of our exploration. Here the model is usually the static image of the original ritual gesture and the reciprocal gestures other participants have added.

Stage two: The dynamisation

The dynamising of a technique is the process we go through in order to undertake our exploration, the various steps and variations we apply to the original model; when we dynamise an image, we bring it to life, it is no longer a static image.

◎ See *Games for Actors and Non-Actors.*

9 Rituals and masks◎

Rituals impose masks of behaviour on all of us. We don a particular mask to face a particular ritual. In recognising these masks we can try to break the rituals.

◎ Ibid.

10 The multiple image of oppression◎

Many images of oppression are created by members of the group and then they are dynamised all at the same time to observe their influence on each other. Sometimes the solutions to our problems are to be found outside our images and not inside.

◎ Ibid.

11 Multiple images of happiness◎

The participants make multiple images of happiness, taking up their preferred positions in the images. Then the effect of these images being dynamised is observed: what does happiness look like? Is one person's idea of happiness compatible with someone else's? Does one person's happiness depend on another's unhappiness?

More often than not we know what oppresses us, what we want to get rid of, but much more seldom do we know what we really want. We must have dreams. Not the sort of dreams that are a substitute for reality but dreams that can help us to imagine the future.

12 The rotating image

This technique is described in full in the 'Screen Image', which is presented later in this book (see p. 170). Essentially it is a means of investigating a scene by rotating characters and spectators; each character or spectator portrays an image of protagonist and antagonist as they have perceived them, and the model is reimprovised with each permutation.

13 The image of transition[◎]

First the group makes the 'real' image of the problem, then the 'ideal' image – how the group would like reality to be. Then, returning to the 'real' image, each participant tries to show the 'image of transition': how it may be possible to go from the first to the second. This is a debate: people can disagree with one another.

◎ See Games for Actors and Non-Actors.

14 The image of the group[◎]

The same technique can be applied to the image of a group. First, individuals make images of how they perceive the group, placing themselves in the image as themselves. Then they can construct an ideal image of the group: how they would like it to be. Finally they attempt to enact the transition from how it is now to how they would like it to be. The same process can be applied to synthetic images of the group.

◎ Ibid.

15 Rashomon

This technique is based on the Akira Kurosawa film of the same name, in which the story of a rape is told from five points of view – that of the rapist, the victim, witnesses, etc. It is particularly useful when analysing a scene with several people, all of whom may have different visions of what is happening.

Stage one: the improvisation

A normal improvisation, cast and directed by the protagonist who has told the story. This can be a scene with a number of characters; anything up to five works well.

Stage two: the protagonist's images

The protagonist makes and positions images of the characters in the scene as she perceived them. Having placed these images, she also makes and positions her image of herself in relation to them. These are subjective images, which can be deformed, extreme, allegorical, symbolic, whatever, and can play with shape, size, distance between characters, positions – everything. There should be no attempt to reproduce the scene as it was naturalistically played.

Stage three: the reimprovisation

The scene is reimprovised, following the basic script and outlines of the original improvisation, with the addition of any elements which arise naturally from the masks. The characters are in fixed images; movement around the stage is possible, but without losing the essential elements of each image. The voices, actions and expressions of the characters are all mediated, translated, through the images. This is how the protagonist perceived the scene.

Stage four: the other characters make their images and reimprovise

In the same way as the protagonist has just done, in succession, each of the remaining characters in the scene makes images of how they felt their character perceived the other characters, once again placing themselves in the image as well. With each new set of images, the scene is reimprovised.

THE PRACTICE

At a workshop in Britain in 1994, a young Asian woman showed a scene of going with her white boyfriend to his parents' home, for the first time. In the original improvisation it is all slightly awkward, but appears generally polite; the boyfriend's parents are uncertain about Asian people, nervous of making a mistake, suspicious of cultural difference, not as warm as they might be.

In the protagonist's image, the boyfriend is hiding some distance away from the table, with his back to everyone and his hands over his ears. The father is an ogre, towering over the Asian protagonist, peering at her; the mother is keeping her distance, arms outstretched in self-protection, as if afraid she might catch something. Other versions were equally revealing; in the father's version, the mother was kneeling, making the sign of the cross, the Asian woman was standing with a leg wrapped around the boy-friend, like some predatory Indian goddess, while the father himself was standing 'on guard', protective of his family, his arms outstretched like a colonial pioneer in the British Raj, ready to fight the 'natives' as soon as he can see the whites of their eyes.

This can be used as a rehearsal technique for any kind of theatre; like the Image of the Group technique, it can also be used for the analysis of a group, particularly if the group seems to have difficulty functioning in certain regular situations, such as meetings. It enables people to see how other people are seeing them.

2 THE INTROSPECTIVE TECHNIQUES

1 The image of the antagonist

This technique is applicable only to the study of a relationship between two people. If the situation the protagonist wishes to analyse also involves other characters, in order to be able to study it in the light of this technique, all the interrelations must be concentrated on the principal conflict, protagonist versus antagonist.

Stage one: the image of oneself

If we have a single protagonist, the group concentrates on the analysis of the problem and the situation he presents. But this technique can equally well be used in the fair mode, with four or five protagonists; we then concentrate on the simultaneous study of each individual, and also on the group represented by these protagonists. We present here the version in the fair mode, the process being the same, somewhat simplified, when it revolves around a single protagonist.

The group chooses a theme, for example love, jealousy or indecision. When I work with a group for the first time, I often propose 'fear' as a theme, because I believe it is fear that makes us accept oppression. A man without fear can be eliminated, assassinated, but never oppressed. The story is told that Che Guevara, under arrest, wounded and disarmed, was treated with disrespect by an officer of the Bolivian army. Without hesitation, he spat in the officer's face. Even disarmed and imprisoned, Che Guevara felt no fear; surrounded by his enemies, he did not lack courage. A short time later, he was murdered. Those of us able to demonstrate such a degree of heroism are indeed rare. Not being heroes, we are afraid. For fear of losing our jobs, we submit to unacceptable conditions of work. For fear of losing a person's love or company, we accept unacceptable situations. Out of fear of death, we accept ways of life we don't like. We are afraid, always; sometimes more, sometimes less. We are conscious of fear, to a greater or lesser extent, or not at all. But fear is always present, on the lookout, conditioning our actions and reactions, conditioning our lives.

Let us suppose that 'fear' is the theme chosen. The director gets the participants into a circle, facing outwards, standing a little distance apart from each other. In this position they must think of a situation involving themselves and an antagonist, of whom they are afraid. The situation must be concrete and very clear: a face-to-face confrontation. The participants must be encouraged to think not in vague terms about fear of society, for example, but of the particular fear that one of its representatives arouses in them. In this work, 'metaphysical fears' will not serve the purpose; we need 'social fears'. The fear must not remain abstract; it must be incarnated in an actual particular person.

As soon as a participant has thought of a concrete, social situation involving her fear, she must translate it into *an image* of her body in the presence of an antagonist opposite her. She can then turn into the circle, but without yet showing her image. When all the participants are turned into the circle, the director asks them to show their images, all at the same time. The images must all be realised at the same time, to avoid the possibility of reciprocal influence.

Stage two: the constitution of families of images

The participants remain in a circle forming their images. The director asks them then to move closer to images similar to their own, keeping away from different images. Thus small groups of image families are formed. Three, four, even five families can be constituted, but it is advisable not to exceed this number so that the participants' attention will not be too divided.

Stage three: the choice of images

The director asks the whole group to choose one image from each family, not the 'best' – this is not a competition – but one which, to a degree, contains all the other images of the same family, symbolising or synthesising them. The chosen image must contain most of the perceptible elements present in the family in its entirety. This choice will always be subjective, guided by the group's sensibility.

In this fashion, the whole group chooses one image representing each family. These three, four or five images will be the synthesis of the images of the fears of the group, on that particular day and at that particular moment.

Stage four: the dynamisation

This stage is relatively long. It should unfold phase by phase in the following order:

1 The director asks the images to place themselves in front of the group, which makes observations on what it sees. These commentaries, even when contradictory, should be limited to simple exposure: we do not engage in a full-scale discussion, since the goal is not to arrive at a specific conclusion. Each person simply reveals their feelings in relation to the images, while the director draws the group's attention to objective details: for example the image is standing or sitting, its hands are doing this, its eyes are turned towards such and such a thing (or not), the body is in such and such a position. . . . With this technique – as indeed with all the other techniques – the task is not to interpret, but *to see what we are looking at.*

2 The director asks the actor-images to give their images a repetitive movement which, by means of its *rhythm*, slow or fast, will amplify their feelings in relation to this particular instance of their fear.

3 The director asks the actor-images to add to their rhythmic images one or more phrases which constitute part of the thought of their characters at that particular moment. The first time round, they must all utter their phrases simultaneously, in order to avoid possible reciprocal influences. They then speak them one by one, so that the whole group may witness them. Thus we have *image, rhythm* and *phrase.*

4 At this point, the director asks each protagonist to carry out a *metamorphosis.* The protagonist has presented to us a particular image, with a particular rhythm, speaking this particular phrase and not another, because, at that moment, a real, concrete moment, she has in front of her a particular antagonist. What image does she have of that antagonist? The protagonist must then, very slowly, metamorphose her image into that of the antagonist, and we see how, little by little, each person transforms themselves into the image of their oppressor.

5 The director asks each actor-image to give a repetitive rhythmic movement to their image of the antagonist, and then to utter one or more phrases which are part of that antagonist's thoughts at that moment. The actors must seek concrete thoughts, not generalities or abstractions.

So, having seen the images of the protagonists with their rhythms and phrases, now we see the images of the antagonists, with their rhythms and their phrases, the whole being the work of the oppressed representing the fears of the group, symbolised or synthesised in these few images.

Stage five: identification or recognition

The director asks who in the group *identifies* with one or other of the images of oppressors – this is a rare eventuality – or *recognises* them. Whoever identifies with one of these images, or recognises it – because he has recognised in it someone concrete, who has caused or is causing him suffering, or because it reminds him of his own antagonist – must replace the actor in this image of the antagonist. The protagonist, who created the image, returns to her original image, the image of the oppressed. When all the antagonists have been replaced, we are left with between three and five couples, each made up of protagonist and antagonist, oppressed and oppressor. The oppressed-protagonists will be able to identify these characters traced from the images they produced, will recognise them, will know who they are, which will enable them to live their parts in the improvisation that follows.

The actors in each couple place themselves opposite one another, and we are ready for the sixth stage.

Stage six: improvisations in two modes

The director gives four instructions, in succession:

1 'Image!' Face to face, the participants take up their respective images of protagonist and antagonist.
2 'Rhythm!' They add the rhythm to their images.
3 'Phrase!' They speak and repeat the phrases they spoke before.
4 'Action!' The couples begin to improvise the scene, simultaneously, in the fair mode. They know only the scene's starting point, since here the idea is not to reproduce the scene experienced in the past, but to undertake an experiment for the future. The protagonist is to try to free herself from the oppression and the fear and the antagonist is to try to show, in action, how this oppressor, the oppressor he knows, would act.

During this stage, one thing almost always crops up, an event which the participants take for a problem but which, in fact, is not one. The actor incarnating the antagonist has a personal frame of reference towards that antagonist: someone he knows, someone out of his own experience, his own life, someone concrete, *similar* to the oppressor who has inspired the protagonist. He knows a *similar* oppressor, but not the same one. So there is already a greater or lesser degree of difference between the antagonist as imagined by the two actors. The protagonist might perhaps have been thinking of her 'father', while the actor incarnating this 'father' (without knowing it), might have been thinking of the sergeant from his barracks. Out of this results an apparent cross-purpose, a surrealist scene, in which one actor calls out: 'Father!' and the other replies 'Soldier!' In reality, the actor-antagonist will merely have detached the 'sergeant' character from the 'father' image. Images are polysemic: therein lies their richness. We must not deprive ourselves of this richness by designating them as incoherent, in the name of a superficial realism or out of a desire for verisimilitude.

The actors must be warned of the possibility of these differences so that it does not distract them in their improvisation. On the contrary, if such differences arise, they will enable the participants more fully to explore the scene, the situation, the protagonists, their fears and our own.

Because it is extremely intense and conflictual, after a few minutes this technique usually sets off an explosive confrontation in which the actors have a tendency to concentrate more on the violence of the activity on stage than on the dramatic action. The director should then suggest the *softly softly* mode. The actors, charged up by this first section of free improvisation, will be open to an enhanced creativity and will learn more about their interrelations.

Stage seven: the second improvisation

After a few minutes, the director interrupts these improvisations and solicits other participants to replace the first group of antagonists, to try using fresh forms of oppression, not present in the first improvisations. The protagonist is thus confronted by a new *weapon* or a new *strategy* from the arsenal of the oppressor. Here 'surrealism' can also take place, though a false surrealism since, in fact, it is simply another real dimension of the first image. The person who originally was the 'father', and then became the 'sergeant', can now become the 'teacher' or the 'priest' or the 'elder brother' or the 'boss' or any other character issuing from the experience of the replacing actor, still incarnating the image of the antagonist.

This second improvisation is also done in both the *normal* and the *softly softly* modes. A third and a fourth improvisation can be done, as long as there are still participants recognising other characteristics of the same antagonist, and offering themselves to test the possibilities of these new confrontations on stage. A multiplicity of replacements of the antagonist is especially recommended when there is a single protagonist. In such a case, we can also put the protagonist in the hot seat, and after several improvisations on one theme, restart the technique with other emotions, other ideas; no technique need necessarily end when all the listed steps have been performed, and not all the steps have to be performed if some seem superfluous to the particular case – the technique should be adapted to suit the person's needs, not vice versa.

Stage eight: the exchange of ideas

The director leads the discussion, an exchange of opinions and impressions, a recap of everything the participants have felt.

THE PRACTICE: FEAR OF THE VOID

In Geneva, we were working with this technique when a young woman said to me:

> 'It's impossible, I can't make an image of fear, since I have no concrete fears. All my fears are abstract.'

I rejected this statement and insisted that she elaborate on some of her 'abstract' fears. She spoke of the fear of death, fear of the future, fear of the infinite, and finally she said:

> 'But it is emptiness which frightens me most.'

I asked her to make an image of emptiness.

> 'I can't. Emptiness is emptiness. Emptiness is something which doesn't exist. How can I make an image of something which doesn't exist?'

'Then make the image of something which doesn't exist but which you would like to see exist. Make the image of this thing, or this person, whichever is the case.'

'No. I still prefer the image of emptiness. . . .'

'But, you just said you couldn't do it.'

'I can try. . . .'

She got onto the sill of the window which, happily, was not very high up:

'You see? For me, that is emptiness.'

'What "that"? It is far from empty out there; there is a park and trees, people passing by, there is the very ground they are walking on. There is no emptiness out there. . . .'

'I'm not concerned with what's outside. The emptiness is right here, in this room.'

I contradicted her:

'Emptiness – in here? But we are here, there are chairs here, tables, objects. The room is full. Perhaps we are not the people you would like to see here, but we are here.'

'That's it. You are not the people I would like to see here.'

'OK. Then, if we are not the person you would like to see here', said I, passing without premeditation from the plural to the singular, 'I suggest you make the image of that person.'

She hesitated for a moment, then took a young man who was seated, placed him a couple of metres away from her, turning his back towards her, and returned to her position on the windowsill.

'See? He is the image of emptiness.'

'Possibly. But it could also be that he is the image of something you want which is far from you. It could be that the image of emptiness is this actual emptiness, the gap which separates you from him.'

'Perhaps.'

'You have made a real image. It is as it is, but it is not as you would like it to be. I suggest you make the ideal image: how would you like it to be?'

She got down from the window, pulled the young man to her side and climbed onto him, piggyback.

'Is that your ideal image?'

'Yes.'

'Then let us go back to the real image.'

She got back up onto the window sill, the young man moved away from her, turning his back, and the image of emptiness reappeared.

'So, your image of emptiness is your wish to ride piggyback on the back of the young man – against his will, since he does not want to be ridden piggyback on. Here the conflict of wills is clear, simpler than "I cannot make an image of emptiness, since emptiness doesn't exist." What does not exist is his willingness to let you do to him all that you want to do to him. We can work perfectly well with this image, just as we would have done with another image, an image which you would call "more concrete". This one is quite concrete enough.'

And, during the realisation of this technique, we were quite able to analyse the relationships of this young woman, who wanted to ride piggyback on young men who did not want to be ridden piggyback on. Her image served just as well as another, more realistic, image would have done.

2 The analytical image

The analytical image is one of the most intense and most complex techniques of the arsenal of the Theatre of the Oppressed. It should not be used if the protagonist does not feel genuinely ready to make use of it; nor should it be used unless the protagonist is familiar with all its stages in depth. Neither must she be under any obligation to go through all these stages; she can stop during the sequence, at whatever point seems most appropriate to her.

Stage one: the improvisation

A normal improvisation – the protagonist chooses the actors who must endeavour to live their characters along the lines she has given.

This technique is most effective when the situation involves only two characters: protagonist and antagonist. It is also useful for working on a situation where the protagonist does not have a clear understanding of what is happening, a situation which gives rise to a certain confusion, or a situation where the protagonist does not know what she wants.

Stage two: the formation of images

The group must let itself be stimulated by the improvisation, but participants must not react like spectators, like consumers, laughing and applauding. On the contrary, they must preserve the most absolute silence and let themselves enter into the mood of *spect-actors*, to be ready to intervene. They must let themselves be assailed by the stimuli of the scene so that these give shape to their bodies and inform their sensibilities.

At the end of the improvisation, the spectators are invited to make images of what they experienced – first of the way the protagonist acted, and then the same for the antagonist. The images should be the product of the perception of a hidden detail, something dissimulated, in the behaviour of one or other character, a detail which, in the case of the protagonist, weakens her, makes her more vulnerable, and in the case of the antagonist reveals his weapons. It might be that the scene has shown a situation in which the oppressed–oppressor relationship is not clearly exposed, where the complexity bears the imprint of confusion. In such a case, the images should show things which, though hidden, were discernible to the participants.

The images should not be realistic, since it will be of no interest to reproduce what we have already seen. The images must show what was visible only to each individual participant because he has put himself into a state of *sym*pathy with the protagonist or the antagonist, with whom he has identified or whom he has recognised. The images can be metaphorical, pleonastic, surrealistic, expressionistic, magnified, deformed – they can be anything, provided they are *real, true, felt*.

To achieve a rich application of the technique, it is advisable to have five images of the two characters.

Stage three: the formation of couples

When all the images have been made, each actor-image seeks her complement in one of the images of the opposite group. Thus we have couples of complementary images. The combination of complementary images is, if you like, random, since the choice is guided more by sensation than by objective reason.

Stage four: the reimprovisations

Once the couples have been formed, each couple is given a relatively short time in which to reimprovise the scene. The actors absolutely must preserve the form of the image as it was originally shown; for instance, if in one of the images we saw the protagonist in the stance of a boxer, the actor is obliged to maintain this stance throughout the whole improvisation. He can move about, but he cannot modify the image in any of its essentials; the image has the function of a filter, since everything that the actor said is decoded by this image: a magnified visualisation of any element of the comportment of protagonist or antagonist.

In the reimprovisations, the actors may say not only what was said during the original improvisation, but also anything they believe to be consistent with what has been said, or anything they believe to have been the subtext, the interior monologue of the characters. These reimprovisations should mix the remembered and the imaginary.

The protagonist and the antagonist witness the reimprovisations.

Stage five: the protagonist takes over the images

At the end of the reimprovisations, the couples return to the stage for a further improvisation in which, each in turn, they must replay as closely as possible the words, gestures and movements of their first improvisation. The protagonist, who witnessed the first improvisation, this time places herself beside her image, and repeats, like an echo, all the actor-image says and does.

The actor-image has created a magnified image, has been 'mimetised' by a single detail, one element, any one aspect of the protagonist's behaviour. Now the reverse happens: the protagonist is to be 'mimetised' by this image, arising from the original mimetism. So she herself will 'mimetise' what she has provoked in the spect-actor. She will magnify a behaviour attributed to her, and the detail will transform the whole, as if she was making a caricature of herself; but this is not exactly caricature, since caricature normally exaggerates what is already evident and here we are magnifying something that was hidden.

After a moment, the director says 'Come out!' and the actor-image comes out of the scene, leaving the protagonist alone opposite the actor-image of the antagonist. For the time being, it is imperative that the protagonist stay with the same image and play out the scene behaving in a manner identical to that of the actor-image she is replacing. After a moment, the director will say: 'You may change!' The protagonist can then, if she is happy with this image, keep it and follow through the improvisation. But if on the other hand she believes that this image is not conducive to her, because it weakens her in her struggle against the antagonist, she can execute a slow *metamorphosis*, transforming herself into a very different image, one which, to her mind, might be more useful in the confrontation – an image of herself as she would like to be.

The process is repeated with all the image couples.

Stage six: the protagonist pits herself against all the images of the antagonist simultaneously

The protagonist comes back onto the stage, but, this time, she must pit herself against all the images of the antagonist. The images of the antagonist all improvise simultaneously, as if they were one person since, in reality, they are different aspects of a single person, the antagonist, fruits of the participating group's analysis.

The images can all talk at the same time, but never with each other. The protagonist can relate to them all at the same time, as if they were a single person, or choose one image and relate only to it. In either case, at the end of this part of the sequence, the director gives the protagonist a potted history of her movements, her certainties and hesitations, during her conflict with one or other image. The movement of the protagonist's body is a writing.

Stage seven: the antagonist pits himself against all the images of the protagonist simultaneously

The actor-image of the antagonist pits himself against the images of the protagonist, under the same terms as described above. The protagonist must observe the scene, trying to discern clearly which images weaken him and how, which images make him stronger and why they have that effect.

Stage eight: further improvisation

The protagonist and the antagonist improvise the scene again, but if the original scene *told the story of an oppression*, now the protagonist must *try to break this oppression* with the help of the images she has seen and experienced. The actors who created the images judged by the protagonist to be prejudicial to her conduct, must place themselves within hearing distance. It is their job to warn the protagonist each time they see her 'backsliding' into these images. They warn her with a sound, of the 'uh-oh!' kind. The protagonist, thus informed of her 'backsliding', must try to execute the same metamorphosis described in stage five.

Stage nine: the exchange of ideas

The director coordinates an exchange of impressions and observations between all the participants.

THE PRACTICE: IN THEATRE, EVEN LIES ARE TRUE

In October 1987, in Cologne, Christian proposed a scene featuring an encounter between him and his girlfriend. He told us that they were always arguing and that he had never managed to work out why. We did *the analytical image.*

In the initial improvisation, we were struck by the fact that the two lovers almost never looked at one other. They talked without looking at each other; neither was including the other. They were 50 centimetres apart, sometimes even closer, but they would not see each other. The absence of the other's body was so complete that they might as well have been talking on the telephone.

At the end of the improvisation, the group made five images of each character. First, the images of Christian:

1 Christian as a 'Red Indian' in a western, dancing, chanting to the sky, circling his girlfriend as if she was a campfire;
2 Christian as a marble statue, standing on a plinth, arms raised, gazing towards the sky, in the attitude of a man who sees himself as handsome, elegant, heroic;

3 Christian like a sulky child, a crybaby, holding on to his mother's skirts, sucking his thumb;
4 Christian ferocious, pointing two accusing fingers at the world to blame for all his troubles. Christian, the innocent counsel for the prosecution;
5 Christian, sick, tired, seated on the ground, hand on stomach, sad.

Then we saw the images of his girlfriend:

1 the girlfriend at the window, looking out;
2 the girlfriend seated on a chair, legs apart, back turned to Christian;
3 the girlfriend smiling at Christian, but without looking at him;
4 the girlfriend in tears, seated on the ground in a corner of the room;
5 the girlfriend masturbating.

We then moved on to the formation of the couples. Here are the combinations spontaneously arrived at:

1 Christian the Red Indian, singing and dancing around his girlfriend seated in the chair with her legs open; though not looking at her, he was preparing to eat her, while she, though in danger, was awaiting a saviour, someone else;
2 Christian the statue played the scene (in fact there hardly was a scene) with a girlfriend who was gazing into the distance out of the window;
3 baby Christian and his laughing girlfriend, mocking him;
4 the ferocious Christian, the counsel for the prosecution pointing fingers, in front of the masturbating girlfriend;
5 Christian, tired and sick, on the floor in one corner of the room, his girlfriend, in tears, in another corner of the room.

Christian seemed fascinated by the improvisations which followed, with the notable exception of the last, in which he took hardly any interest, preferring to look at other friends in the group. Even the third, which we found difficult to bear, he watched with great jollity, I would even say with content. But the one that aroused the greatest enthusiasm in him was the scene in which he was shown as an Indian, the very one in which, more clearly than in any other, he wouldn't set eyes on his girlfriend.

Then came the moment when Christian had to assume each of these five images in turn and preserve or abandon them as he wished. Not only did he not abandon a single one of them, but he exaggerated them all, as soon as their original actors left the stage. He reached paroxysms of exaggeration, orgasmic extremes, in his images of the Red Indian, the statue, the baby, the counsel for the prosecution. It was not even funny yet, paradoxically, he seemed to want to make us laugh. To his despair, perhaps, we did not laugh. On the contrary, we were awaiting, in trepidation, the fifth improvisation, the one in which Christian had to be the image of himself tired and sick: if he followed through the logic of this exaggeration, he must surely die. . . . But no: Christian exaggerated an extroverted fatigue, an operatic sickness; it was touch and go whether he would break into an aria from *La Traviata*.

At the end, he asked, 'So, how did you like it?' as if we were in a normal theatre, after the opening night of a play in which he was playing the lead.

> 'It's up to you to say . . . you improvised the scene, not us. How did you like it? Tell us what you liked and what you didn't.'

Christian answered that he had liked it all, because it was all true, he really was like that, even more so, so much so that 'even we' had been unable to see it.

> 'You are all this? Even the last image?'

> 'Even more so. . . .'

Sabine protested. According to her, Christian had been lying throughout.

> 'He wanted to put on a show. . . . To play a scene for us. That is not him. . . . When the rest of us improvise a scene, we throw ourselves completely into the scene, we upset ourselves, we expose ourselves, we reveal ourselves. Not Christian. He lies non-stop, he just pretends. In my view, I don't think it would be possible to work on that scene, it would be pointless.'

She was furious.

Everything that Sabine was saying was true, but it was not the whole truth. It is true that it was very difficult for us, given Christian's histrionic fury, to understand the relationship with his girlfriend. Even the actress who was playing her had said that he had given her so little by way of information or direction that she believed that, for that reason, her performance could not be considered valid. She did not know who the girlfriend was because he himself did not know.

> 'I don't believe it,' I said. 'If he gave you so little of any value, it is very possible that he gives even less to his girlfriend.'

It is true that Christian was living his own personality, while the actress was playing a personality based on someone she did not know. But the pair of them there, in front of us, were living and animating an improvisation. It is true that Christian 'was lying' all the time, if one can call his histrionics lying. He was lying, yes, but *it is true that he was lying.* Letting our perceptions be clouded by the lie prevented us from seeing the liar in action. If, however, we had taken notice of him, we would have seen the liar Christian in the action of lying. Christian 'was putting on a show': he *truly* was telling some lies.

It is possible that the five images of Christian may have been inspired by the lies he had told us, verbally or in the original improvisation. It is possible that he was not truly as he had shown himself to us. But it is true that he wanted us to think him thus.

If he was lying, this implied somewhere the existence of a truth. The liar not only wants to make the false pass for the true, he also wants to hide a truth.

What truth?

> 'I know I am like that, but I don't want to be any other way, I want to stay as I am. I am like that with my girlfriend and with everybody. If I was ever to change, we would end up splitting up. What we want is to argue with each other, together, to be close to each other so that we can not look at each other. So?'

Christian could not stop talking, defiant because he wanted to prevent us believing him. So?

So? So nothing, everything was fine. What we could discern in his discourse was excess, plethora, extreme intensity; in short, what he wanted to make us see. And if he said that he was like that because he wanted to be like that, OK then, let him be like that; we could do nothing else. At best, we could suggest that he try, simply for the experience, playing the scene of their relationship in a more tranquil, less anguished fashion. I even suggested that they improvise the scene once again. Christian refused: 'I'm very tired.' I pushed. 'No, I really don't want to. Actually I feel a bit ill. . .' and he went and sat alone in a corner of the room.

There was no longer anybody in the other corner: the actress-girlfriend was sitting on the floor, with the rest of the group. After a fashion, they were reproducing the fifth couple.

In theatre, the problem is not one of knowing whether someone is lying or telling the truth: the problem is seeing that someone is in the process of doing something, of acting. For, even if the protagonist is lying, the action of lying is always true.

3 The circuit of rituals and masks

If it is true that the rituals of daily life force each of us to don the appropriate, adequate mask, that is to say, a mask whose function is to cushion the collisions between people and the actions they are called on to carry out, or obliged to carry out, then equally it must be true that the refusal to avail oneself of this mask, or the use of an inadequate mask, will explode the ritual, or considerably modify it, or even reveal its inadequacy. In fact, a struggle rages between the ritual and the person, and the mask is the result of this struggle.

Stage one: the ritualised improvisations

The protagonist constructs several different scenes. Four or five is a good number: fewer than four renders the technique less effective, more than five makes it confusing. Each scene must be 'placed' in a different space in the room. The protagonist must play herself in the improvisation of each scene and she must instruct the other actors on its essential elements. The actors, while retaining their freedom to improvise, must follow these basic directions. The protagonist must choose scenes that contain different oppressions and in which her own behaviour is to some extent different, specific to each scene. For instance, the protagonist will surely have different ways of conducting herself with her boyfriend, her analyst, her father and the grocer at the corner shop.

Each improvisation should last several minutes, after which the director asks the observing group how the protagonist has evolved in the scene, what her most striking characteristics were, what the nature of her mask was. The spect-actors should show their observations with their bodies, rather than expressing them in words. If a number of spect-actors have shown a number of images, after they have all been seen the group must choose a single image for each scene. Before each scene, the director must ask the protagonist what she *wants* from each of the other characters, so that the protagonist will exercise herself to get what she wants, so that she will take action instead of simply showing herself 'the way she is'. I insist on this point: a character is an action and not a reaction, a verb and not a noun, at bottom there is always an 'I want'. We can adjectivise her but she must not adjectivise herself. The actor must love and *we* may then say of her that the character is a lover. She must not show the lover: she must show a character in the act of loving.

Once the first ritual scene is finished, the protagonist moves on to the second, while the actors of the first 'de-activate' themselves while staying in the playing space of their scene. The second scene is activated and improvised for a few minutes, after which the director asks the group a few questions on the principal and specific characteristics of the protagonist in her mask for the second improvisation; and, as always, the responses should be offered in the form of performance or image rather than in words. We proceed in the same manner with the third, fourth and fifth improvisations.

Stage two: strengthening the mask

After this first series of improvisations, the director makes a list of the characteristics of the protagonist (her *masks*) as remembered by the group for each ritual scene. Next, he asks the protagonist to do the sequence of scenes again, in the same order, trying in each case to exaggerate and to magnify these noted characteristics. Where the protagonist had shown signs of big-heartedness, she must be even more generous; where she had been intolerant, she should push intolerance to the extreme; where she had been violent, let her excel in violence.

Stage three: the conflict between the masks and the rituals

Next the director asks the protagonist to improvise one scene with the magnified mask corresponding to that scene and then, retaining that mask, to go and improvise in all the other scenes for which the mask is, on the face of it, inadequate. The other actors in the scenes must react in conformity with this new behaviour by the protagonist. We will thus be able to deduce 'what would happen if. . . '.

In one workshop, we had a protagonist on the psychoanalyst's couch, sucking his thumb in a state of regression. Then, thumb still in mouth, he went off to meet his girlfriend. He then discovered that his attitude did not simplify the situation. If he harboured this 'thumb in mouth' behaviour in secret, symbolically he still carried it with him in most of his relations with other people. That was the way he was; he discovered that even if he never ostensibly displayed this attitude to his girlfriend, in fact it was 'as if. . . '. In another workshop, a protagonist was disco dancing with her girlfriends in a state of wild abandon. With the same extroversion, she rejoined her parents or went to work in a restaurant, or busied herself with her children. With the parents, the children and the customers this mask of joy and extroversion improved their relationships. But her magnified mask of despondency with its 'atmosphere of Juliet's tomb' – the mask of her relationship with her parents – stopped the *élan* of the disco band dead in its tracks.

This technique allows the protagonist to see that being one, he is multiple. Rare indeed are those people who are always and everywhere the same as themselves. We transform ourselves and, sometimes, we do it to adapt ourselves to a ritual which constrains us, which limits us, which prohibits our expression of ourselves. In these cases, something is not working and that something is either in us or in the ritual. To change it, we first have to see it, theatrically, aesthetically.

4 The image of chaos

This technique is very similar to the Circuit of Rituals and Masks. It gains from being used straight after the Image of the Hour. Here, we must see the protagonist at different moments in his life, where his attention is more or less solicited or exercised; moments of greater or lesser energy, of more or less intense interest, of greater or lesser pleasure or grief, moments of certainty or of confusion. By means of *the image of chaos*, the protagonist tries to see this disparity and to correct or restructure whatever he believes requires modification.

Stage one: the formation of images

The protagonist tries to show five images (or more) of himself in five (or more) different situations of the day, situations in which he behaves in five different manners, goes in five different directions, has five different forms of energy. He constructs, one by one, images which show himself and his antagonist in each of these five moments; these two characters are then immediately replaced by two other actors, each time. The five scenes are improvised at the same time, in softly softly mode.

Stage two: the fair

The protagonist promenades between the scenes, which are being improvised simultaneously. For each scene, there will be between three and five rounds of improvisation, each of two to three minutes' duration. After each round, the protagonist gives some instructions to the actors, to modify their behaviour in directions which, he believes, will harmonise his image between these different scenes. If he judges it necessary, he can, in the last round, replace each of the actors-protagonists in a lightning forum, the better to make explicit and put into practice his idea of the ideal scene.

Stage three: the discussion

The discussion should focus on what occurred in the different rounds, and especially on the participation of the protagonist in each of the scenes and the greater or less intense interest he was able to bring to one or the other scene.

5 The image of the 'cops in the head' and their antibodies[⊚]

® This technique is most applicable to scenes in which the protagonist wants to do something, but, for reasons he may or may not understand, fails to do it. There are no concrete 'cops' present, stopping him doing it, but still he doesn't do it; so there may be 'cops in the head' instead (A.J.).

Stage one: the improvisation

The protagonist improvises the original scene with the actors he needs.

Stage two: the formation of images

The director asks the protagonist to sculpt images of the 'cops' which were present in his memory or in his imagination during this first improvisation, using the bodies of participants not involved in the improvisation. These images must represent concrete people, real, known, familiar people. Not abstractions like 'the family', but the father, the mother, the aunt; not 'society' but the cop, the boss, the lawyer; not 'the Church' but this particular priest, and so on. These characters were not visible to us when the improvisation was taking place, but they were present in the head of the protagonist; these are characters which inspire in him – or are in their origins – fears, desires, phobias, vexations; characters who have come to his mind, with greater or lesser intensity, during the improvisation.

Next, the director asks the participants if they have spotted other 'cops' in the protagonist's head, or if the improvisation has awoken 'cops' in their own heads. If they have, they must make images of these cops. Obviously if the participants have seen them, it is only because they themselves are familiar with these particular cops in their own heads, and because they have established a *sym*pathetic rapport with the protagonist. The protagonist has the right to accept or refuse these images. He does not accept them unless they awaken in him a precise memory of a particular person; cops are concrete individuals, people we know.

Stage three: the arrangement of the constellation

The director asks the protagonist to arrange these 'statues' in a sort of constellation, in which the latter will occupy the central position. What is the relationship of each 'statue' to him? How far away from him is each 'statue' positioned? Is it facing in or out? Standing or seated? In front of him, opposite him, behind him, perceptible but only out of the corner of his eye? Is it unbearably close to him, or desperately far away? And what are the inter-relationships of the statues? Can the invisible characters (the 'cops') see each other, or, by contrast, are they hiding? Are there conflicts between them or are they united?

Before setting out on the next stage, the director must draw the group's attention to the objective details of this constellation: the details of each 'statue' and the details of the structure of the constellation, the space in which the visible characters (those of the improvisation) and the invisible ones (the 'cops') are situated. She should make observations on the relationship between the protagonist and these figures. The director must always speak in her own name, and should stimulate the protagonist and the other participants to speak similarly for themselves and express their observations, even when these are contradictory. We should not seek to resolve the contradictions, but to throw light on them. We must always try to see the images from an objective point of view and to distinguish this objectivity (that which is indisputable: the person in the image is either sitting or standing) from projections ('My impression is that she is frightened', 'It seems to me that he is in love', and so on.) Anything can be said, as long as attention is always paid to the distinction between 'it is' and 'it seems to me', between that which exists without me and that which depends on my perception.

Stage four: the in-formation of the images

This is one of the most beautiful stages of this technique, perhaps because it is one of the most theatrical and most moving phases. The director asks the protagonist to approach, in whatever order he chooses, each of the *images of the invisible characters* of the constellation, and tell them, slowly and in a clear but low voice, something which refers to the common past of the protagonist and the person represented by this image. Each 'conversation' must start with the phrase 'You remember when. . .' and close with 'and that is why. . . '. That is to say: the 'conversation' must evoke a real event that occurred between the two of them, or was witnessed by both of them, and which had consequences; for instance: 'Dad, do you remember that day when you beat me with your belt? That is why I realised that you are a weak man. . . .' The actor embodying the image must not show his reactions. He must stay like a waxwork, like a photo, inanimate. On to this 'statue' the protagonist projects his memories and his emotions. The actor, who when he was 'sculpted' was 'formed', is now 'informed'. With this form and this information, he will be able to live his character in the stage which follows.

Thus, to each one of them, the protagonist will tell his memories, his emotions, his fears, his desires, his complaints. The other participants must maintain an absolute silence while this is taking place: these are secrets which the protagonist is revealing to us, and to which we must, all of us, be sympathetic witnesses, in solidarity. These monologues of the protagonist with each image are revelatory, and these revelations must be received without applause or censure.

Stage five: the reimprovisation with the images

The director proposes that the scene be reimprovised.

The antagonist(s) are instructed to do whatever is necessary to work towards the goal of making the scene end in the same way as it ended in the improvisation. The protagonist, on the other hand, must try to change the scene in line with his desires.

While this improvisation between protagonist and antagonist develops in a purely realistic style (as it might happen in reality), on a second level of play the images of the invisible characters also start to improvise, but in their case the style can be surrealistic, since they are not part of the visible reality. The images can utter any thoughts that come into their heads, motivated as they are by their form and by the information supplied by the protagonist, and also, obviously, by their own sensibility, their intelligence, their own lived experience. But – and this is very important – the images *cannot move around*. They must talk in a low, distant tone, but must be audible to the protagonist. Only the protagonist can move them; he can do what he wants with them and they will offer no resistance. *But they will not obey.* For instance: the gesture 'Go away!' will have no practical consequences on the image: the protagonist has to physically move them away, and if they are removed in this fashion, they should have a built-in tendency (if they are well motivated) to return to their initial positions, in slow motion. All the images always come back in slow motion, to their original positions.

So we will then have two levels of play: one, realistic, the arena in which actors and protagonist operate; another, surrealistic, the arena of protagonist and *images*. The protagonist is the only person living in both levels, the actors and the images being incapable of dialogue with each other.

The director must use her sensitivity to judge how much time the protagonist needs to try to free himself from these phantoms without becoming totally worn out. It is particularly stressful for the protagonist to play on these two levels, in two different styles, to live in these two levels as if he was simultaneously living two stories. What is more, he sees that, in spite of all his efforts, *the ghosts always have a tendency to come back to their places and to repeat the same things*, just as, indeed, they do in real life. This tension is difficult to live with, it demands great emotional gymnasticism and requires a huge effort from the protagonist. It is incumbent on the director to guard against this effort exceeding reasonable bounds and thus becoming ineffective.

Stage six: the lightning forum

The director organises a lightning forum: she asks all the participants, or as many as are willing, to line up and, one after another, go on stage, replace the protagonist and try, for a minute or so at most, to carry out an action which they think might be effective against the *ghosts*. The protagonist observes the interventions. By virtue of its rapidity, the lightning forum has the advantage of allowing interventions from all the spect-actors and obliging them to get straight to the point. It also allows the protagonist to see a variety of finished or sketched solutions, good and bad, more or less successful, a whole gamut of thoughts, sensations and opinions.

The lightning forum over, the director asks the protagonist to take up his position on stage once again.

Stage seven: the creation of antibodies

During this section, the protagonist lives only on the level of the 'cops', the surreal level. And on this level, armed with his own opinions and desires, but also fortified by the suggestions gained in the lightning forum, he will try to *show the participants* the way he believes each 'cop' can be disarmed. As his intention is to *show*, he will fight the cop in a magnified, demonstrative manner. As soon as anyone in the audience has understood the tack he is taking, his actions and his arguments, that person immediately replaces the protagonist in his combat against that particular 'cop' and the protagonist can move on to a second 'cop'. The cop he has just dealt with and the person who replaced the protagonist can then wait together on the sidelines until the next stage; or they can just carry on improvising. The same happens with the second 'cop', and so on until all the 'cops' have their *antibodies* in front of them.

At this point, the scene will have exploded into various subscenes, each featuring a 'cop' and an antibody, both partners being free to develop, starting from their original form and information, whole characters living a complex situation.

Stage eight: the fair[a]

The director must stimulate both parties to increase the tension and the creativity within each of these different and simultaneous scenes. If they wish, they can spend a moment or two preparing their separate scenes, and then all are invited back to improvise simultaneously, in the fair mode. The director invites the protagonist to wander around the 'fair', spending more or less time observing each scene, each combat, according to his interest. The movements of the protagonist during his promenade are a *writing*. This writing must be *read*, and the director will then recount it to the participants in the course of the following stage. The participants may disagree about this reading, since here we are using a *multiple mirror of the gaze of others*.

Stage nine: the discussion

The director and the whole group exchange ideas, but without attempting to arrive at consensus or to win arguments. It is important that the participants *admire* (wonder at) the protagonist's actions and reactions, and that they reveal their *surprise*; it is equally important for the protagonist to *admire himself in the midst of these admirations*. The protagonist is not here to be judged, but *to surprise himself with the surprises* that he brings to light.

To an even greater extent than in the other techniques of the Theatre of the Oppressed, in the image of the cop in the head surprise and admiration are essential elements in the acquisition of knowledge. To surprise oneself means to learn something new, something strange, something unusual about oneself: something possible!

THE PRACTICE

Vera's friends

I started to use and develop this technique in the workshops I do every year with my group in Paris. Vera told us a story and

[a] As has been stressed before, the director should vary the steps according to the particular case; not all the steps will always be necessary, or other steps, other dynamisations, will sometimes seem more appropriate. For instance, in this technique it may sometimes be more effective to see each improvisation that makes up the fair separately, rather than all together. In a such case the participants in each image may spend more time preparing, telling each other the stories which led to them intervening (as cop or antibody) and then enacting one of these stories (A.J.).

improvised the scene: she had just separated from her husband and the scene took place at her workplace when she was joining her colleagues for a coffee-break. Usually, Vera's colleagues were good colleagues. But that day, the first time that they had got together since Vera's separation, things had changed.

A male colleague, Jean, started off with some jokes in dubious taste and ended up offering, as cool as a cucumber, to replace Vera's husband in her bed. Not every day, but whenever she needed him and he felt in good form. He spoke to her like a tradesman offering his services: 'Women need it, and a friend in need is a friend indeed.' Simple, no?

Françoise would not stop going on about how sorry she felt for abandoned women – without listening to Vera, who was telling her over and over that she was the one who had walked out, as she couldn't take it any more. Françoise was in full flood of pity about the situation: she wanted to share the pain, the terrible sorrow, which in fact was completely non-existent.

Marie-Jose, her boss, marked Vera down for it. For her, the group itself was diminished by having a divorcee in its midst.

The jokes were just as unbearable as the outright aggression, and Vera proposed that we analyse the scene in Forum Theatre form. We tried.

We tried, but it wasn't working. Not that the scene was not stimulating; on the contrary, it was wonderful to see how the actors let their 'Loch Nesses'® emerge, and revealed that anti-feminist ideology, full of prejudices, which we call *la France profonde* (the real France). The forum did not work because the situation seemed impossible to resolve. There was nothing to be done. All the women who went on stage and replaced Vera ended up, sooner or later, throwing in the job – in the scene – or leaving the stage – our job – when they were not choosing straightforward physical violence or *magic solutions.*®

It was then that I understood that it was pointless to do a forum, since Vera was entering the scene already defeated: she was effectively experiencing a scene of aggression, a scene in which no further possibilities exist. Vera was defeated even before the coffee-break, when she was on her own. Then – and this is how this technique came into being – I asked her to speak in mono-logue. For a few minutes, Vera spoke all alone. Then, as in a delirium, she began a dialogue with the dramatis personae of her day-to-day life, characters invisible to us: her father, her mother, her brothers, her neighbours. We listened to everything she was

® Loch Ness: a reference to the mythical monster which, as legend has it, inhabits a stretch of water in Scotland called Loch Ness; occasional 'sightings' usually only feature the neck and head of the animal, most of its body remaining under water. Boal gives the name *Loch Ness* to the thoughts, the deeper desires, of oppressor characters, inclinations which are usually hidden, because of the social function of these characters or their obligation to keep them in check – in a good forum these concealed urges should rise to the surface; the monster should be sighted (A.J.).

® In Forum Theatre an intervention is said to be magic when, in order for it to succeed, it changes the givens of the reality. An extreme example might be an intervener taking the place of a penniless, jobless person and miraculously finding £10,000 in the gutter. As with everything in forum, it is up to the audience to decide what is magic and what is not (A.J.).

saying to these immaterial beings, people she alone could see in front of her. I asked her then to make the effort to show us these interlocutors. The monologue went on: Vera was in front of the mirror, trying to make herself look pretty; but now the invisible 'cops' were there, telling her when it was not acceptable for a married woman to separate, telling her how worthless she was, how she was becoming a prostitute, a woman of the streets, etc. It may be that all these family figures had never talked to her in this way, but that was how they were thinking and perhaps they had said these things apropos of another woman. The fact is that Vera retained the memory of these familial condemnations. Marvelling, we saw the coincidence: everything that her friends were thinking, saying and doing during the coffee-break was part and parcel of the thoughts, the moral values, the judgements which already inhabited Vera's mind: these were 'cops' preparing the way for the external aggressions, preventing Vera from expressing her own thoughts, since they were there, firmly lodged, expressing theirs. To everything her real friends were saying, the 'cops in the head' were answering: 'She's right, that's it exactly, divorcees are worthless.'

Vera had not been beaten by the visible antagonists – which in all honesty would have been pretty ridiculous for a modern French woman living in Paris. The reason for her defeat was herself and the waxworks museum, the cemetery, she carried around in her head: her embalmed cops.

A little boy, Henrique's friend

Henrique made the image of his 'cops' but among them he placed a protector. It went like this: in the initial improvisation, Henrique showed a scene in which he was asking his sister to lend him money. He needed a lot: 2,000 *cruzados*.◉ His sister was rich, she loved him a lot; in principle she had the means to lend him this money. Henrique constructed several images. In all of them, someone was accusing him of being a good-for-nothing, an 'artist' (it should be said that Henrique was an actor). These were very aggressive images. But, amongst them, he placed a very gentle, very sweet image: the image of an intimidated little boy, seated on the ground, represented by the gentlest, sweetest participant in the group.

During the fifth stage, the entrusting of the secret recollections,

◉ Since this was written the Brazilian currency has changed its name and been devalued at least four times. With Brazilian inflation running at 70 per cent a month at that time, it is not possible to know what exact sum of money this 2,000 cruzados represented. So let us take the author's word for it: a lot (A.J.).

Henrique recalled to each one the aggression they had subjected him to. But to the little boy he said:

> 'You remember, that evening, many many years ago. . . ? It was raining cats and dogs, and we were alone in the house and we were scared of the lightning. That's why, whenever I am afraid, I remember you.'

Throughout the improvisation, Henrique never let go of the little boy. When I asked him to construct *antibodies*, he created them for all the 'cops', but not for the little boy. Right through all the various stages, he showed himself incapable of asking his sister for all the money he needed, and ended up settling for a tenth of it. Finally, he left the stage, taking the child with him. I asked him:

> 'And what about that image – don't you want to create an antibody for it?'
>
> 'No.'
>
> 'Why?'
>
> 'Because he is me.'

The 'old' Joachim and the phagocyte 'cop'

⊚ Phagocyte (Gk. φαγο-eating, devouring): a leucocyte (or white blood corpuscle, lymph-corpuscle) which under certain conditions has the power of absorbing or destroying pathogenic microbes by a process of intracellular digestion, thus guarding against infection (OED). Boal is clearly reverting to the Greek root here, as his phagocyte is not always a beneficial agent (A.J.).

Nuremberg, October 1988: Joachim told us a love story. He was in love with Clara, a woman twenty years his junior, who seemed to love him. But the two of them were not seeing each other, not talking to each other, except on odd occasions and always when surrounded by other people. He was a lecturer, she was a student, and they met at the faculty, in the midst of the other lecturers and students. When they did meet, they would talk work – studies, problems in the faculty, strikes. . . . They loved each other, but never touched on matters of intimacy. They knew that they loved each other, but neither was sure of the other's love.

One day, completely by chance, they met in a bar. This was the scene which Joachim recounted to us. At the faculty, they used to talk in a very animated fashion. In this bar, by contrast, they hardly talked at all, each waiting for the other to say something. And, as they waited, all they said was:

> 'What?'
>
> 'Were you going to say something?'

'I didn't understand what you were saying. . . .'

'You were saying?'

And that was it. Then they said goodbye to each other and each went back to their own place, ruminating on all the unspoken words, all the unexpressed desires.

Joachim improvised the scene. Then I asked him to construct the image of the 'cops' lodged in his head. Here they are:

1 a young man lying between Joachim and Clara on the table, laughing and making fun of them;
2 a boy, snivelling;
3 a severe man, looking at him and pointing a finger at the fourth image;
4 a man who was engaged in some intellectual pursuit, reading and writing.

I asked Joachim, 'Are there only men?'

'Nothing but men,' he answered, quick as a shot.

I asked the participants if they had seen other 'cops' in Joachim's head, making it clear to them, however, that they could only have seen them if they, themselves, had these particular 'cops' in their own heads. The images started to appear, but Joachim spurned them: he would not recognise a single one. Someone showed the image of an old woman looking at Clara with a hard-faced inscrutable gaze.

'Yes . . . perhaps . . . I think that that could go in,' he said, without enthusiasm.

Then came a double image, a very beautiful image, which greatly moved us: a female participant formed first the image of a young woman, with a smiling, gentle face, her legs and arms open – and next, behind this young woman, she placed another woman who, using her arms and a tablecloth found in the room, was completely hiding the face of the first. The two together formed a single contradictory image: the open legs and arms of the first woman preserved the gentleness of the image, though her face was hidden, while the face of the second woman was a mask of obscenity, emitting an expression of mockery or impertinence. Unhesitating, vehement, Joachim said: 'That's it! That's dead right!'

Someone remarked that we were dealing with a 'phagocyte cop': the woman with the mocking smile had 'phagocyted', devoured and digested, the face of the soft and gentle woman, creating a monster whose head tormented its body.

'That's it exactly, a "phagocyte cop".'

And Joachim went on, fascinated:

'Look at her, she's eating the other woman up, she's already eaten the head, soon she'll eat the body. . . .'

I stopped him in mid-flow and asked him to move on to the following stage, in which he would have to talk to the images. He started with the image of the little boy, and reminded him of moments in his own childhood, his solitary tears in vain, the tears of a lonely child shut in his room. In front of the severe man, he reminded him of paternal recriminations about his schoolwork. To the young man seated, he recalled a very poor colleague, who was studying twenty-four hours a day. To the woman he recalled the recriminations of his mother. Then he sat down and, faced with the impossibility of talking to the woman with the hidden face, he stayed put, in front of the 'mocker', asking her: 'Should I believe what you seem to be, this front you put up? Why are you lying?'

During the fifth stage, Joachim remained seated, immobile, carrying on the conversation with the Clara actress as in the first improvisation. That preoccupied me: he had reacted to nothing, had changed nothing. When I then proposed the lightning forum to him, Joachim answered that it would not be necessary.

'Why?' I asked.

'Because I already know what I have to do. . . .'

This seemed pretty strange to me: he said he knew what to do, but he was doing absolutely nothing. Anyway, I acceded to his demand, since for me the people, the participants, are more important than the techniques, the latter being at the service of the former rather than vice versa. I then suggested to Joachim that he create the antibodies. He answered, 'Okay, but in my own way. . . .'

'His own way' was as curious as could be. He began by gathering the characters back together, asked the boy-actress to cry louder, more strongly and more violently. She obeyed, he took her by the arm and led her in front of the woman with the inscrutable look. He made the 'little boy' enfold the woman in her arms, told her to cry even more loudly and strongly, to hug the woman even more violently in her arms. The actress obeyed, accommodatingly. The poor woman made her face even more impassive, but then lost all her aggression and went on to the defensive, alarmed by the child's screams and tantrums: she tried to calm the 'little boy' down.

Next, Joachim took the accusing man by the arm and led him over to the studious young man. The man continued to give orders: 'Do your homework!' And the young man studied away. The one cancelled out the other, just like the woman and the child in the first pair of images.

Joachim did not concern himself any more with these four characters, who were cancelling each other out. He laughed, watching them. Then he got his breath back and defaced the monster. If previously he had put the four ghosts into pairs, now he did the opposite: he tore the tablecloth from the face of the young seated woman with her legs and arms open, and, for the first time, he saw her face. Having cut the chain which tied them to each other, he moved the mocking woman away, pushed her into a corner of the room, came back to the young seated woman, laid her down and lay down beside her. The young woman enfolded him in her arms and the two of them stayed there, lying down, watching the mocking woman, who was ill at ease and did not know what to do. After a moment, Joachim took Clara, who was seated at the counter of the bar, and placed her next to him, himself lying between these two women as if they made up a single woman. Very similar in aspect, the two women did, in fact, form a homogeneous whole.

I waited to see what was going to happen. I had thought of continuing through the stages of the technique, but Joachim was following his own path. And so much the better. He asked: 'Can I do it over again?' 'Certainly,' said I, and the actors took up their original positions again.

Joachim did the same things with the same gestures. Almost. For, when pushing the snivelling child against the woman with the inscrutable look, he demanded: 'Go on! Eat her! Bite her! Chew her up!' The poor woman was worried about this cannibalism, but she held fast. 'Bite! Eat! Take a bite out of her!' continued Joachim, euphoric.

Next, for the severe man/studious student pair, he became a coach:

'Don't answer, let him get angry. Say nothing, don't look at him!'

Seeing which, the man got angry for real, and Joachim, happy and excited as a football supporter, urged on the studious young man even more:

'Chew him up, kill him, eat him, devour him!'

Over-excited, in complete contrast to his usual demeanour, Joachim raised his voice. Some participants were laughing at this, but gently. We all wanted to see where this would end. Joachim turned to the 'monster' pair. The mocking woman gave vent to a cry of comic fear:

'Okay, I'm going of my own accord!' and she ran into a corner of the room.

Joachim then sat down beside the young girl with open legs and arms. Very tenderly, she enfolded him in her arms and legs. Clara approached and held him from behind, tenderly. And, for a moment, they stayed like that, the three of them together on the floor. As for me, I said nothing. Finally, Joachim spoke:

> 'I know that in reality things aren't like this. But they are like this. They are and they aren't. . . .'

> 'Like this in what way?'

> 'When I look at Clara, I see that other woman there and I hear these men. . . . I have discovered an important thing: I have many cops in my head, many. I have some who order me to work all day long, others who tell me that I am getting old, others who put me on the defensive against this or that – all in all, all sorts of cops. My head is a veritable police barracks. It contains even more cops than those you have seen. But I have discovered an important thing: some of these cops are phagocytes, some have the capacity to eat others. They are cannibals and some of these cannibals have a serious appetite. What I need to discover is which are the good cannibals and which need to be eaten. . . .'

The group laughed a lot. And Joachim, after close consideration, asked me:

> 'Do you believe in the existence of a cannibal "cop in the head"?'

> 'I believe in everything, my dear Joachim, everything.'

I believe in everything . . . especially in theatre. And I believe in all the things which, thanks to theatre, can be spoken and heard.

OBSERVATIONS

1 This technique presents a difficulty. The protagonist tends to place his 'cops' around him, neglecting the advantages of, and the values innate in, a constellation. The director must insist that the protagonist make use of distance and perspective, and of arrangements of different heights; so that he organises the 'cops' according to their respective affinities and repulsions, instead of simply placing them side by side, like a wall. One should not accept such a 'wall of cops' unless the protagonist constructs it, not inadvertently, but expressly, on purpose. We are involved in making theatre, so we need to use the aesthetic space which is there; if it is not used, it becomes an empty space, which also has a meaning.

2 The 'cop' is not necessarily an image with a gun in his hand or a finger in the air. He can also present himself in a seductive guise. We define as 'cop' the image present in our heads, at a point of action, which obliges us to do what we don't want to do or prevents us from doing what we do want to do. Its presence means that our desire is diluted and that, instead of enacting our own desire, we enact the 'cop's'. This can come about by violence or by seduction, by toughness or gentleness, by word or by gesture, with audacity or timidity.

3 On occasion – and this enriches the process – the protagonist places in his *constellation*, not only his own 'cops in the head' but also the 'cops in the heads of his cops'. These very rich *constellations* have a tendency towards confusion. In such cases, it is necessary to use the *softly softly* mode in order to obtain a clearer vision of the conflicts.

4 All the techniques presented in this book are *aesthetic* techniques, that is, sensory, artistic techniques. Sometimes, some participants quite simply want to verbalise their thoughts, or illustrate them with fairly obvious images. However, an image should not be the mere illustration of a word or a phrase. In these cases, the best thing to do is to enunciate that word or phrase. An image must be constructed, created, in an aesthetic climate, a climate of sensations, emotions, sounds and movements, and not uniquely in the medium of words.

5 Frequently, during the fifth stage of this technique, the protagonist spends the best part of his time and energy struggling against his 'cops', paying little attention to the antagonist. Almost always, this is revealing what is happening in reality:

we occupy ourselves more with our interdicts than with our desires. But it may be that the protagonist is acting in this manner in order 'not to see' the real antagonists. The theatre stage is intimidating. The director should watch out for this, and be ready to help the protagonist to look around. But, if he insists on expending his energies exclusively on his 'cops', then this should be taken not as an accident but as a sign.

6 The image of the 'cops in the heads' of the spectators

This technique is identical to the preceding one. It involves the same stages, except that here the spect-actors intervene from the very outset, constructing the images of their own 'cops in the head'. These projections may be made by identification, recognition or resonance.

Almost without fail, the protagonist recognises as his own images shown by the participants, quite simply because, almost always, *sym*pathy arises.

7 The image of the rainbow of desire

No sensation, emotion or desire exists in a pure state in the human being. Even that love so pure between Romeo and Juliet is not exempt from aggression or resentment. Love and hate, sadness and joy, cowardice and courage, mix and mingle in constantly differing proportions. That which emerges socially, at any given moment, is only the 'dominant' (strain)® of all these forces at work in the human soul.

This technique helps to clarify these desires, these wills, emotions, sensations. It allows the protagonist to see herself not as a univocal being, like her physical image reflected in a physical mirror, but as a multiple being, her image reflected by the prism which is the other participants. The protagonist's passions appear here in all their colours – invisible to the naked eye – in the same motion as when the white light of the sun, passing through rain, mutates into a rainbow in which we see all the colours the white light concealed. To the phrase 'as clear as daylight' we counter: 'No, as dark as daylight, which lies – as clear as the rainbow, which tells us the truth.'

® For clarification of Boal's use of the term 'dominant' in reference to wills and counter-wills, analogous to its use in musicology, see *Games for Actors and Non-Actors*, London: Routledge, 1992, pp. 57–9.

As stated before, the sequence of steps in this technique is not immutable, nor need every stage be executed if it does not seem appropriate. Suit the technique to the person.

Stage one: the improvisation

The technique opens with an improvisation 'scripted' and 'directed' by the protagonist. So we have a person-personality who lives the part of the protagonist and person-*personnages* (characters) who bring the antagonists to life.

Stage two: the rainbow

The director asks the protagonist to create images of her desires, of her states of mind, loves and hates, fears and fortitudes, in short of all the forces she feels are at work and of importance in the scene we are to study. The protagonist shows these images with her own body. They are then reproduced by participants who identify with them, or recognise them, or participants in whom the images have triggered a strong resonance. The participants who reproduce the images must be doing it not simply in acceptance of the roles, but because they really wish to incarnate them.

When the protagonist has perfected this sculpture of images and is satisfied with them, the director asks the rest of the participants if they want to suggest others. If so, each must show his image with his own body, and the protagonist can accept or refuse them. She must be able to say of them: 'I am like that' or 'That is a part of me', since the aim is to achieve images that reveal characteristics of the protagonist; we are no longer dealing with 'cops in the head', which are the desires of others, but with the desires of the protagonist herself.

Stage three: the brief monologues, the confidences

The director asks the images to place themselves 'on the side-lines', as on a football pitch, outside the playing area. He asks the protagonist to utter, in front of each image and directed to it alone, a brief confidential monologue, which must begin with a phrase along the lines of 'I am like that because. . .' or 'That's not the way I would like to be, but I recognise it because. . .', or even:

'I would like to be much more like that, because. . . .' She must always refer back to what she really thinks and feels. She must reveal how she feels on discovering the way she is. The actor-images will use this information the better to live their parts in the improvisations that follow (while still using imagination and not just memory) since, though they may use words and movements in that part of the sequence, they may not undo the essential elements of their images; the image should not be lost, because it works as a 'filter' of what is said.

The confidences must be imparted in front of all the participants, who have the function of witnesses.

Stage four: the part takes over the whole

The antagonist returns to the stage and the protagonist sends on the images, in whatever order she wants, for whatever reasons. Each image has around one minute to confront the antagonist, alone, as if that image on its own was the protagonist in her entirety, as if the part was the whole, as if the rainbow had only one colour. The group observes the effects of this monochromatic combat, its consequences, the paths this relationship could take.

The protagonist sends the images on one by one, to do battle 'on the pitch', and as soon as the director feels that the scene is sufficiently clear, he sends them back 'to the sidelines'. The antagonist should react as if he was dealing with different characters or else as if a single character was suddenly changing his behaviour – since each colour that comes on stage takes up the scene exactly where the previous colour left off. When all the images have been through this first 'round' of their combat, we move on to the following stage.

Stage five: the whole rainbow

The protagonist sends the images, one by one, back onto the pitch, but this time they stay there. As they are constituent parts of the protagonist, she cannot ignore them, feign their non-existence, but she can control them or, at least, try to control them. Thus she arranges them, one at a time, in a sort of constellation, with the antagonist as its centre, and she moves them around at will, placing them closer to or further from the antagonist, facing him, sideways on, or back to him, as prominent or unobtrusive as she likes. By this means, the protagonist can determine the proportionate impact of the characteristics that animate each image. For instance, if she thinks that an image is too violent, she can move it further away, placing it in such a way that its aggression is less striking. It must continue its relationship to the antagonist, as if it was alone with him. The antagonist confronts all the images as if they were a single person: the protagonist.

Variation

The protagonist can make two constellations: first, as above, the rainbow as she perceives it, in the status quo; second, the rainbow as she would like it to be, ideally. The similarities and differences can then be noted; or we can see the rainbow move in slow motion from one configuration to the other.

Here there are at least two points, of equal importance, worthy of note:

1 The movements of the protagonist in her placing of the images on stage, her resolution or indecision, her hesitations or certainties, are, in themselves, a writing to be 'read', confronted and discussed with the protagonist and the other participants in the group. When the protagonist is on stage organising her rainbow, she loses sight of herself and cannot observe herself. It is useful for her to be told how she conducted herself during the placing of her images.

2 The behaviour of the antagonist in relation to each image is also a series of signifiers: how would he have behaved if the protagonist was only like this or only like that? In the improvisation, when he faces the protagonist, he faces a whole; now that he sees her in detail, he must choose which (singular or plural) of these 'colours' he needs or wishes or prefers to establish a relationship with, and how.

It is also worth noting that the signifiers in both cases (and throughout this process) are not absolute or rigid containers of meaning – they are polysemic; depending on who reads them, their signification will be different – another rainbow. So all that is being offered by the group is observations of these signifiers, which can lead to speculations about their meaning.

Stage six: will versus desire

The protagonist is instructed to move from one image to another in her 'real' constellation (as opposed to her 'ideal' constellation, if that variation has been used), engaging in a one-to-one dialogue with each 'colour'. Each colour is one of the protagonist's *desires*, which may or may not concur with her *will*; the will is a conscious decision, the desires are amoral forces. So in this section we try to reconcile will and desire.

The protagonist initiates the dialogue with each desire with a phrase along the lines of either 'I would like to be more like that because. . . ' or 'I would rather be less like that because. . . .' The conscious will addresses each of the (often unconscious) desires and tries to convince them to be more or less like they are. If the protagonist wants to magnify a desire, she and the desire discuss how to achieve this; if she wants to minimise a desire, she argues with it to try and persuade it to change accordingly. But whatever the protagonist's goal, to minimise or maximise, *the desires, being amoral and unresponsive to reason, must inevitably become magnified in the course of the dialogue*, either because of the supportive stimulus of the will's persuasion or hardening in self-defence, in argumentative response to the will's contradictory stance.

The protagonist spends a short time conversing with each colour, then moves on to the next (either of her own accord or at the urging of the director). In the process the colours, the desires, all become stronger.

Here again, the choices, the order, the time taken with each colour and the tenor of each encounter – all of these are a writing to be read by the group.

Stage seven: the protagonist takes the antagonist's place

When the protagonist has organised her *constellation*, her rainbow, and has 'charged up' each desire as above, the director asks her to place herself at the antagonist's side, or behind him. She will thus be able to observe and to experience the rainbow of her desire from the same perspective as the antagonist. When we talk to someone we know what we are saying, but we have very little idea of how it is understood. Equally, when we carry out an action, we know what we are doing, but we do not know how our action has been perceived, felt or experienced. In this new perspective, the protagonist will be able to see how she is seen, to perceive how she is perceived.

After a moment, the director asks the antagonist to leave, with the protagonist remaining in his place. The images must follow through the scene as if nothing had changed.

Stage eight: the agora of desires

The director then asks the protagonist to leave the playing area. Left on their own, the images then begin *the agora of desires*: each image, until now unaware of the others, can debate, engage in dialogue with the others, take action in relation to them. The issue in hand, the confrontation with the antagonist, must continue to be addressed.

Initially, each desire is to seek out its complement, the most contradictory desire, to do battle with them; if two desires home in on one desire, the latter has the choice of which to conduct a dialogue with. The pairs thus established make a little space for themselves and converse, trying to really understand these desires, from the heart and from the brain. After a time, the director instructs them to 'Change desires' and other pairs are formed in the same way. After sufficient of those dialogues, they are instructed to change for a third time.

At least three such sets of pairings should take place, but it is vital that, even for a brief moment, each image recognise the existence of the others and establish a relationship with each of them. We must be able to sense and to examine the relations between most or all of the images, two by two. Afterwards, they can do what they want, *à deux*, or all together.

During the agora, the protagonist can circulate freely around the performance space, the better to see and hear the alternatives, the opinions, the solutions; another writing.

Stage nine: the reimprovisation

Very quickly, the desires are dismissed and the original scene between protagonist and antagonist is reimprovised. The protagonist is instructed this time to try to make her will prevail. The outcome of the scene may or may not be different.

Stage ten: the discussion

All the actors must tell of what they felt or noticed from within the scene, while the other participants express what they felt or noticed observing the scene.

The director must coordinate the discussion, without ever trying to 'interpret' or 'discover the truth'. He must only signal the originalities, the curiosities, all the aesthetic aspects of each intervention – the signifiers, rather than the signifieds.

THE PRACTICE

Soledad's sensory images

In Rio de Janeiro in May 1989 Soledad told how, after ten years of marriage, she had decided to separate from her husband. According to her story, her husband, a soft, slow fellow, usually incapable of taking a decision, had decided to refuse the separation. Soledad loved her husband a lot, but could not bear his slowness. She left the family home and communicated her decision by phone. The husband, wounded, accepted this – at least, he accepted on the phone; in fact he accepted without accepting, just as he had refused while not refusing, said things while meaning the opposite, and did not really know what he meant or wanted.

As Soledad was definitely quitting the house to go and live alone, they arranged a rendezvous so that she could move out what belonged to her. This was the scene which Soledad offered us.

Soledad enters the house, which appears to be deserted, and discovers her husband in their bedroom, lying on the bed, eyes closed, listening to music on a Walkman. She calls him, touches him, nudges him, until, finally, he becomes aware of her presence. She starts putting her clothes on one side, while the husband continues listening to his music. She sorts through her books. The husband is still listening to the music, but now has his eyes open and is spying on all his future ex-wife's movements. Soledad then tells him she is going to take her records. The husband protests, contests this, forbids it: the records are all mixed up, he no longer knows which records belong to whom. She is the one who wanted the separation, let her take the consequences. One of these consequences is to lose her records, since the records 'live' in this house which belonged to both of them. That's how he sees things. Soledad kicks up a fuss; it is useless. She explains her reasons, but he does not accept or understand them. Soledad looks at her husband, who is lying there listening to his music and saying no to her. And the scene ends there.

I asked Soledad to make the rainbow of her desires. She began. The most notable characteristic of her construction of the images was the time she took and the minute detail with which she arranged each image in relation to her husband. Here are the images:

1 Soledad in bed, lying beside her husband, holding his hand; later, when talking to the image, she reminded him of times they had when they lived together, happily.
2 Soledad seated on the bed, explaining, like a tender mother to her delinquent son, that the husband should not behave like that: 'You are like a baby, glued to its mother's nipple. . . .'
3 Soledad pushing her husband out of the house, forcing him to move, to act, to do something. Later, in action, the actress-image cried out: 'Do something, hold me, don't let me leave!'
4 Soledad the child, kneeling on the bed, hands joined, imploring: 'Look at me!'
5 Soledad trying to strangle her husband in hand-to-hand combat.
6 Soledad sadistic, showing how she would rip the covers off the records and break them into pieces. This gave her immense pleasure. She wanted to issue threats – an activity which gave her pleasure – but was not carrying them out. Her pleasure resided in threatening and in seeing the fear in her husband's face: 'The records are the only sensitive part of your body: watch – I am tearing you to pieces, I am smashing you. . . .' Soledad explained later that making him suffer, frightening him, gave her pleasure. A pleasure which was almost literally orgasmic. 'If he had allowed me to take the records, perhaps I might not have done so.'

At the rainbow stage, when the colours confronted the antagonist, first one at a time then all together, it was the strength of the physical relationship that each colour established with the husband that most touched us. Either Soledad was caressing him tenderly, or else, tenderly, body to body, she was pushing him out of the room and out of the house. The scenes all ended up on the bed, in a sort of test of bodily strength. We especially noted the scene with the husband and Soledad the strangler, in which both of them rolled off the bed and onto the ground, tangled up in the sheets, all of which felt very sensual and free from danger.

> 'It's true. If I had really wanted to kill him, I would not have made the image of a strangler, I would have put in a woman with a gun in her hand.'

She was right. A gunshot, once fired, is irreversible; it kills and it's over. A man cannot put up any bodily defence against a gunshot. It is a cold-blooded death. Strangling, on the other hand, is sensual: of necessity, the two bodies have to be very close to each other, they have to touch. Strangling is gradual: it reaches its peak little by little, always leaving open the possibility of reprieve before arriving at an orgiastic death. What's more, Soledad was not a physically powerful woman, and if it had come to such a test of strength she would probably have been the loser.

But that would have required him to act ... and he – the bastard! – would not do a thing. . . .

Soledad commented:

> 'If I had really wanted to take away the records, I would have gone there at a time when he was not there. I have the keys. I could even have stolen his records, as well as taking my own. But no. I wanted his presence! I could have instructed a removal firm and taken the whole house away . . . I preferred to argue with him. And I ended up taking nothing. . . .'

The frightening love

Zurich, March 1989. Benno, an architect, with his seven-year-old son who will not let him work, who wants to play the whole time. One day, Benno has to finish the plans for a new block of flats, and he is hard at work, leaning over his desk. The son enters; they argue. The scene closes on a prostrate Benno, guilty, since he has succeeded neither in finishing his work nor in playing with his son.

I asked him to make images. Here is his rainbow:

1 The stern father, forceful, laying down the law, maintaining order. Face to face with his son, it's a massacre. The son reacts as if he has a horrible, threatening, paralysing demon in front of him.

2 The father as 'his son's best friend'. Benno drops everything, sends the plans and designs flying, starts playing on the floor. His work will not be delivered the following day.

3 The worker father: the son comes in. The father doesn't even notice his presence, doesn't answer his questions. Of all the images, this is the most wounding for the son: the image which ignores him, which does not identify him, either as son or as human being, the image which nullifies his identity. The son feels voiceless – since he is not being listened to – and body-less – since he is not being seen.

4 The teacher father, who explains at length and with infinite sidetracks, going into minute detail, how the relations between father and son should work, what their respective duties and rights should be, all about salaries, added value and so on. The son falls asleep during the explanations.

5 The victim father: he shows how he suffers from not being able to play with his son as he would like to, from not being understood by his son (who should, however, understand him), from not being understood by anybody in his house or outside it. He shows the son how he suffers such suffering – here a suffering, there a suffering, everywhere a suffering. In short, a father in a state of great anxiety . . . and the son gives up playing: better off alone than in bad company.⊚

⊚ A popular Brazilian saying.

6 The father babies the son, treats him like someone mentally deficient rather than like a child: everything the child does is stupid, and obviously the father doesn't have time for stupidities: come back when you've grown up.

7 His last desire surprised us into laughing out loud. Even Benno laughed. It was the image of the super-loving father, the father for whom the son is the sole *raison d'être* in the world, this beloved, idolised son! The scene had barely got into its stride before the son fled in terror. A love like that would be unbearable, really – it was so over the top.

In constructing his rainbow, Benno placed in front of the son, side by side, the loving father and the father who was laying down the law, and between the three of them he placed the father-companion. In the improvisation that followed the son preferred this composition, the other fathers finding themselves scattered around the room: the worker father visible, in the mid-distance, the teacher father visible but inaudible. The two with whom the son argued the most were the victim father and the father who babied him. The child did not like it at all, and nor did Benno. Which is why he moved them away, placing them close to the touchline. Laughing at himself and a little ashamed, Benno did not even want to see them:

'I was like that, but not any more. That's all in the past.'

'The past how long ago?'

'Yesterday. . . .'

'And yesterday is already the past?'

'Sure, why not? It's just a matter of wanting it.'

And that is what he wanted.

The elephant of Guissen, in West Germany

May 1989. For the first time, I had decided to use a Cop in the Head technique in a public showing, marking the end of a week-long workshop. It is completely normal – and a common enough occurrence – for participants who turn up at the public shows and do not know each other to have a tendency to hide the principal problem that they are experiencing, to mask it, to symbolise it. However, I think that even then this technique can be useful. I believe it was, on this occasion.

So, that evening at Guissen, a woman offered herself as protagonist. She wanted to gain a better understanding of her relationship with her (male) friend. Possibly she offered herself on a spur-of-the-moment whim, since immediately afterwards she seemed indecisive, intimidated in front of the public. Fair enough – from her seat she saw only me; from the stage she saw 200 people.

'So, I have to improvise a scene and show what I believe is going on inside me and what I want from him. Is that it?' she asked, worried.

'Yes, that's it exactly. Theatre is conflict, theatre is about wanting. What do you want?'

'Who, me?'

'Yes, madam, you!'

She hesitated in front of this audience. I offered her the chance to quit and return to her seat, but she wanted to go on; so I carried on asking her what it was she wanted from her boyfriend or husband or lover. Eventually came the answer:

'I want an elephant . . . .'

Of course we all laughed, the audience and I alike. I even thought of asking her to suggest something more 'concrete' than an elephant, but then I thought that an elephant could very well hide many other things. An elephant, even a small one, can hide a lot.

We improvised the scene, and after the first minute the laughter evaporated from the auditorium. We were still seeing a woman asking her friend for an elephant. If we had been paying attention only to these words, doubtless everything she was saying would have seemed absolutely ridiculous. But this woman was passionately set on getting something from this man. We could translate 'elephant' and hear instead 'love', tenderness', 'social position', 'orgasm', 'understanding', 'forgiveness' – so many possibilities! 'Elephant' could mean anything – who knows, maybe even elephant, which was the last thing on our minds. No matter: this woman was asking this man, in desperation, for something he did not want to, or could not, give to her. And the technique was just as useful as if she had asked him for the simplest thing in the world, like, for example, an elephant. . . . And yet, he was refusing.

We also spotted another, more important, thing: she was asking, demanding, but offering nothing in return. Wanting without giving.

In the rainbow she showed us:

1 a child-bride, snivelling, asking for a plaything, tapping her foot, as if she wanted an elephant as a cuddly toy from people who appeared to denote 'daddy' and 'mummy';
2 a terrified spouse, frightened of the dark which concealed a real elephant, immense, furious, with massive, heavy feet like tree-trunks; she was in full flight from her husband (her companion – the man), as she would have fled a troop of carnivorous elephants;
3 a spouse with wounded legs, unable to walk, but unaware of the presence of the husband, having no relationship with him: her only thought was of her mutilated legs. She was not asking for help, she was immersed in self-pity;
4 a boxer-spouse, apparently training and using the husband's

head as a punch-bag. She was not relating at all to the husband, all her attention being concentrated on her arms, her fists; she was happy in her physical superiority to the punch-bag, which could not return her blows;

5 a spouse in front of the mirror, admiring herself, hugging herself; again there was no relationship with the husband. I had the strange sensation that the woman thought of herself as the image in the mirror and not herself;

6 a spouse seated beside an imaginary river, with an imaginary fishing line in hand, pensive, alone, not looking at the husband, hoping that the fish won't rise to the bait;

7 a spouse far removed from the husband, but looking at him and speaking from afar, from far far away, in murmurs, her speech inaudible to him.

Of all these images, only two, the first and the last, preserved a clear relationship with the antagonist, the husband. All the rest were images of self-contemplation, of withdrawal into oneself. To such an extent that the actor playing the antagonist felt a mere spectator: several times he left the playing area and I had to ask him to go back to his place in the improvisation. In fact, in constructing the images, the woman did not concern herself with him. But it is one thing to take no notice of someone who is absent, another to ignore that someone when he is present: the former was a case of her *not including him in the scene*, the latter a case of her *expelling him from the scene*. The husband-actor would come back into the playing area, and I would do my utmost to enable her to see him, drawing her attention to the distances between the various images and the husband. She, knowing full well that the husband was present, would not even look at him. I believe she was distancing herself even from the fact that we were all present, that we were in a theatre. In one of her images she placed herself in front of a mirror; in front of us – and in front of the images – she seemed to be in front of a huge mirror, in which she was gazing at herself, looking at all the images, who were her. And, remember, out of all the possible images, she had chosen the image of the mirror.

She always seemed to be the image, not herself. At least that is what I felt.

Once the rainbow had been formed, I asked her to send in the images, one by one, to engage in dialogue with the husband. Dialogue occurred in the first and last cases. In all the others, the husband had no need even to answer back or say anything whatsoever. Mute, he contemplated the images' monologues, as a spectator. And none of these five images took any notice of him either.

After the dialogues, during the section in which the part takes over the whole, I asked the woman to form a constellation with the colours of her rainbow. The first five images she put on stage she placed in relation to each other but sidelining the husband, who became a sort of satellite of this constellation of five women. Finally, she placed the first image, the snivelling child, between the five women and the husband, and, much further away, the last, the image of the woman talking from such a distance and at such a minimal volume that she could not even have intended to be understood . . . especially in the light of the fact that the other images were speaking at the same time.

These last two images were put in rather as if their positions didn't matter, any old how. I asked her then to place herself at the antagonist's side, the better to appreciate the scene from the husband's point of view.

'My God,' she said, a bit panicked in front of the tableau of images.

Then, breaking all the rules of the game – and without my standing in her way – she remodelled the whole rainbow. First, and without any hesitation, she eliminated the figure of the child. Next, she spent some time looking at the circle of five women, removing them one by one and placing them, like the first, behind the husband, at his back, in such a way that he could not see them, and sufficiently removed from him that he could not hear them. In the way she related to each of the images one detail struck us clearly, visibly, distinctly: the image with the wounded legs she lifted roughly from the ground and pushed around; she made a horrible face at the terrified one, terrifying her even more; the one who was boxing with her punch-bag, she hit round the head; she placed a great big smacker on the lips of the one who was cuddling herself in the mirror; and as for the one who was fishing, she threw her rod into the river. After which, she expelled all five.

Then she returned to the antagonist's side. For a few minutes she just laughed, loud and long. She did this in front of an audience of 200 people, some of whom were laughing, others of whom were trying to guess, or at least to get a sense of, what was going on in the protagonist's mind. After the laughter, she said to us, very soberly: 'It isn't like that. . . .'

At this point the husband and the image were engaged in banal conversation: 'We need to talk, we must understand each other, you take no notice of me,' etc. The 'It isn't like that . . . ' cut this short. 'What is it like then?' asked the image.

The woman got up, and, once again transgressing the rules of the game, took the place of the image. A silence . . . the woman looked at the antagonist in front of her, then looked at a man who was seated in the audience and was accompanying her, looked again at the 'husband' and said, quite simply: 'Let's go!'

Where to? To do what? We will never know, but that is not in the least bit important. All we know is that 'Let's go!' implies a decision by two people. As the announcement of a movement, 'Let's go!' is, in itself, a movement. All the forms of relation which had gone before were about blockage, about self-satisfaction or permanent, insipid lamentation. Even in the last instance, where a dialogue was taking place, the man was virtually extinguished. 'Let's go!' was a departure, a beginning, a new stage: it was an action, a decision. The impossible demand – 'I want an elephant' – had been replaced by a possible proposition – 'Let's go!'

'*You* will give me an elephant' is singular. 'Let *us* go' is plural.

Where to? They alone knew.

In a session of the Theatre of the Oppressed, everything that we learn or discover is aesthetic learning or discovery; we learn and discover through the senses. We learn and discover above all by seeing and hearing. And on this occasion we saw and heard this woman say 'Let's go!' and then go and sit down, laughing, next to the man. Who was he? Only the two of them knew.

Bon voyage!

Linda the lovely

At New York University, in January 1989, Linda told us about an incident. She had worked through the summer in a hotel, and of course was expecting to be paid at the end of the month. Come the end of the month, she sought out the manager to ask him for her pay cheque. She only had half an hour, as her train was leaving at six o'clock. The manager talked, and talked; time was passing, Linda missed her train and it was hard work getting her wages.

She even had to forcefully turn down a 'proposition' from the manager.

We did the rainbow.

1 Linda, pushed for time, wants to catch her train; there isn't another till three hours later; she absolutely must catch this one.
2 A timid Linda, who doesn't know how to deal with money – perhaps at bottom she thinks that she doesn't deserve the money she has earned working as a waitress in the hotel.
3 Timid Linda, fearful of the manager, a powerful, stern-faced figure; this was the first time that she had had to face up to him.
4 A Linda who wants to go back and work in this hotel the following year; she shows herself to be efficient, practical, quick, a real 'little man'.
5 Patient Linda, used to waiting in line; well, that's just the way it goes.
6 Linda on edge, wanting to explode, scream, shout out loud.
7 Linda the seductress. Linda does not bely her Christian name;◉ the manager is a man like all other men – he wants to seduce her; Linda is happy about it, she likes to seduce.

◉ In Portuguese, Linda means beautiful, lovely (A.J.).

In the following stage, Linda sent on all the images she had constructed, one by one. The manager responded in a different manner to each image. Until the seventh: this improvisation ended up in bed, as we might have expected.

Linda then had to make the constellation of her desires around the manager. We all thought that the 'lovely Linda' would be placed a little out of play, at the edge of the stage; the seductress Linda would not be of much use to her if she really wanted to get her cheque and go. Quite the reverse, since the seductress Linda disrupted, contradicted even, the apparent haste that Linda had demonstrated and proclaimed. But, against all expectation, she placed 'lovely Linda' right in front of the manager, highly visible, beside the two timid women. A little further out she put the one who wanted to go back and work in the hotel next year. Then she positioned the patient image with its back turned to the manager and facing the only violent image of the group which, from a considerable distance, remonstrated loudly against the manager, with, however, little chance of being listened to.

We watched the rainbow, her constellation of desires. I insisted that the furious one was much too far away to be 'operational'.

Linda moved her a little, but at the same time brought her closer to the two timid ones, who once again neutralised her.

We observed that the 'patient Linda' was still in the way of the others, who were tripping over her. But Linda left everything as it was: she paid no attention to the patient one and left her there, resigned.

She continued to make adjustments which changed nothing, but showed herself incapable of moving out the 'lovely Linda', who was almost sitting on the manager's lap and was the only really dynamic one, the violent one being too far off. In the end I mentioned this fact, but Linda was not bothered about it:

'I am leaving her where she is.'

I then asked her to place herself at the manager-actor's side, to see what he was seeing. She did so.

'So? What do you see?'

'I see that I really am beautiful . . . .'

In spite of her hurry to catch her train, her need to leave at speed, the fear the manager aroused in her, the fact that she did not feel attracted towards him – in spite of all these things, Linda could not forget that she was beautiful, she could not forgo the pleasure she experienced in seducing.

And there is nothing wrong with that. The only problem was that, as a result of spending all her time trying to seduce, Linda ended up missing her train.

New stages

Two other stages can be added to this technique to make it an extroversion technique.

In Cologne in 1989 I asked Margarethe to go through the whole technique, which she did. Margarethe's partner was not paying enough attention to her. Of herself, she showed images of backing down, with the exception of two: a Margarethe the seductress and a violent Margarethe.

After the agora of desires, I asked her to remove, magically, all the images which did not please her. She left only these two 'active' images, which she liked a lot.

Then I asked her partner to make his rainbow as well. His images were of no interest to Margarethe. In the following stage, I asked Margarethe to play with these images. Curiously, she still took up physical stances similar to those of the images of herself that she liked: the seductress and the aggressive woman. From her point of view, she was winning in every 'round'. At the end she told us:

> 'It was as if, when I removed the images that I didn't like, I was removing them from myself. Then, when I went to do battle with my partner, the only images I was left with were the ones I liked.'

So much the better.

8 The screen-image©

This technique is especially recommended for the study of relations between two people. It goes without saying that the results are even better if the two people are both present.

It is based on the fact that, when we have a relationship with someone, we inevitably project onto that person an image which is not a exact copy of them and which sometimes doesn't even resemble them. It is as if there was a screen between the two characters, on to which each is projecting an image of the other. For instance, the relations between an old couple: each projects on to the other events from the past which perhaps their companion is not even conscious of; or a father–son relationship, where the father still sees his adult son as a child, while the son will always project on to his father images fabricated from memory and imagination.

The screen-image has three main characteristics:

1 It is a *filter*: everything the other person says or does will be 'filtered' by this image we are projecting onto them. All the signifieds will be 'translated' by this filter, thus acquiring a different signification; what we hear is only rarely what has been said; what we see is only rarely what has been shown. The 'filtered' images do not match the images transmitted.

2 It is also a *screen* in the other sense of the word, a physical barrier, like a folding screen; the screen-image does not allow us to see the real image of the other.

3 It is a *shield*; if my interlocutor projects onto me an image, this image, which is not identical to me, may still suit me, I may like it. Since the screen-image is a *screen*, my interlocutor will not

© In some early editions of *Games for Actors and Non-Actors*, by a translator's error (this translator) the title 'Screen Image' is wrongly attributed to a technique which should be called 'Projected Image' (A.J.).

see me; since it is a *shield*, I can, if I want, make use of it. For example, this is what happens with bosses: their underlings project on to them the image of boss, which makes it easier for them to adopt the demeanour of bosses.

Stage one: the improvisation

This is a normal improvisation, as already amply described in the preceding techniques; the protagonist chooses one participant as his antagonist ('antagonist' is merely a technical term here – the two might be lovers, friends, relations, whatever). One or more spect-actors are also chosen as 'witnesses', whose task is to note all that happens through the process. If working with one improvisation in front of a whole group, then the whole group will perform this function, but this technique can also be used with a large group, split into groups of at least five around the room, each doing one story; the five people will be required if going on to *the rotating image* stage (see p. 170).

Stage two: the formation of screen-images

Using a spect-actor, both of the actors in the improvisation sculpt in front of their opposite number their *projected image of this other* – the image as they have seen it – significantly modifying the body of the other in the statue, with the intention of showing what perturbs or afflicts them in the other, what they fear or find threatening in him, what strikes them most forcefully, the thing which makes genuine dialogue impossible.

So in front of the protagonist will be his image as projected by the antagonist, and vice versa, in such a way that neither of the two can see the other. (This is no more nor less than what is happening in real life.)

Stage three: the improvisation with the screen-images

The actors reimprovise the scene in the following manner: when-ever one of them wants to say anything, he must ask the image the other person has projected onto him to say what he wants to say: 'Tell him that. . . '. The screen-image then says, out loud, what it has been asked to say, but keeping its own image characteristics, thus filtering the actor's discourse. Even the voice must be the voice of this mask; so if, for instance, an image is tight-lipped, the voice should be correspondingly tight-lipped – if the image is the image of an ogre, the voice should be an ogre's voice. The screen-image transmits the messages, but, in the act of transmission, it translates them, which transforms them.

The director should allow the improvisation to run long enough for the actors to get used to the technique and to be able to use it effectively. The screen-images are enhanced by this period of improvisation, which enables them to store up information and log suggestions for action.

Stage four: the images become autonomous

The director then gives a signal to the screen-images to become autonomous. The protagonist and the antagonist back away from their images and observe the scene, in which the screen-images, though autonomous, pursue their combat. Everything they say or do must be considered as said or done, and must be taken on board by the protagonist and antagonist when they return to the playing area in the next stage. Using their imagination and their creativity, not limiting themselves to their memory of the original scene, the spect-actors playing the masks should push them to their extremes, taking the scene to the ultimate, logical consequence it would reach if these masks were in control.

Stage five: the protagonist and antagonist return

After a time, the director signals the protagonist and the antagonist to take up their positions again behind their screen-images. At first they are to echo their masks, their screen-images, both bodily and vocally; after a moment, the director asks the images to retire, and protagonist and antagonist are left on their own again. They should keep their image, if proceeding to the rotating image stage, and improvise the scene in that shape.

If not proceeding to the rotating image stage, after a short time they may drop their masks. Then, for the first time, protagonist and antagonist are truly able to see each other. The scene must continue until the damage done by the screen-images has been repaired – if, by any chance, this is possible.

Stage six: the rotating image

This stage is optional. It is less complicated than it sounds; in essence, three participants take the protagonist's place in succession, offering 'advice' on how to approach the antagonist; and three further images of the antagonist are also offered.◉

First of all, the protagonist takes the place of the antagonist, taking up the mask he perceived, the mask he designed for her. The spect-actor who was playing the protagonist's mask, now takes the place of the protagonist, taking up an image of his or her own choice, an image which he or she thinks might be useful in dealing with this antagonist; this is the spect-actor's 'advice' to the protagonist. A short improvisation with these new images takes place, protagonist and antagonist still trying to achieve whatever their original incarnations were trying to achieve.

Then the next rotation takes place. The person who has just played the protagonist now takes the place of the antagonist, taking up the image that she perceived (not literally what she saw, but what she felt) of that antagonist in the original improvisation or in any of the successive improvisations. The person who originally played the antagonist's mask now offers his advice by playing the protagonist in an image he believes would help. Another short improvisation.

The next rotation: the protagonist-replacement now moves on to play the antagonist, as he perceived him, and the original antagonist becomes the third replacement for the protagonist, offering a third idea. A third improvisation.

Each of these three improvisations can pick up where the previous one left off, or they can start afresh each time.

Finally, the original protagonist and antagonist return to their roles. The original protagonist has now seen three ideas of how the relationship might be improved – he can choose any or all or none of these ideas. The scene is reimprovised, the protagonist doing his utmost to achieve the outcome he desires.

◉ The original participants are protagonist (P), antagonist (A), protagonist image (PI) and antagonist image (AI). The four rotations thus run as follows, the first-named always playing protagonist and the second the antagonist: 1) PI v. P; 2) AI v. PI; 3) A v. AI; 4) P v. A.

Stage seven: the exchange of ideas

The witnesses and participants report back to the whole group and the director coordinates an exchange of ideas.

9 Contradictory images of the same people in the same story©

© See also Rashomon, an image/rehearsal technique which explores similar areas.

When we are in dialogue with another person – even when we are face to face with that person, one to one – our dialogue is inhabited by other people, living or dead, who rise up, resuscitate themselves in our memories and deform themselves in our imaginations. The people to whom we refer explicitly in this dialogue, as well as those who surface in it in diluted form, masked, covered by veils or smokescreens, are always present, and they influence our words and our thoughts. But each of these people is always double; and each of these double people is perceived by both one and the other interlocutor. You and I perceive the same person in different forms. This person is, in reality, a third person. But, as the one person is double, when we speak of them, we are not both speaking of the same person. We think that we are saying the same things of the same people when, in reality, we are saying different things about different people. We need at least to be conscious of this, to have an *aesthetic consciousness* of this; we need to see which is which, who is who, what is what.

In this technique the stage that precedes the improvisation is extremely important. The protagonist and antagonist must be given as much time as they need to accomplish it.

Stage one: sensitising the antagonist-actor

This stage is not necessary if the couple presenting themselves wish to use this technique to study a situation of which they have shared experience, as a couple. But if the protagonist is the only one who is living through or has experienced the situation, then she needs time to explain to the actor who will play the antagonist everything he will need in order to be able not only to understand the scene but, above all, to live it. The actor can and must ask questions with a view to enriching his understanding, enhancing his perception of the dialogue as much as possible in depth and complexity.

Only when the antagonist-actor feels intensely and completely sensitised to the improvisation can it begin.

Stage two: the improvisation

This is a normal improvisation.

Stage three: the images

The director asks the two actors to create contradictory images of every person present in the dialogue, whether mentioned or not. The director pronounces, one after another, the names of these people, and the two actors, without watching each other (or, if the space is too small, trying to look at each other as little as possible), sculpt the images of these people, using the whole of the stage space for this task – if necessary the stage space can be enlarged. All the images are placed within the same space, without division between the protagonist's space and the antagonist's space. They both position the two image-statues of each person in whatever form and at whatever distance they have perceived or felt them in relation to themselves and in relation to the other. When this double constellation is finished, the director makes her observations and invites the participants to express themselves freely on everything they have seen; the similarities and differences between each pair of images of a single person mentioned, the distances or proximities, the facial expressions, and so on. As always, the contradictions between the observations must be absolutely respected.

THE PRACTICE

In Berlin, in 1988, Bernardt and Helga, a couple, suggested working on their awakening in the morning. Their problems began there.

Helga, constructing images of the characters she had in her head, placed two women in the space: two woman friends protecting her, defending her against Bernardt. When I asked Bernardt to construct his images, he wanted to use Helga's, taking them as they were. I forbade him:

'These are the images Helga has made.'

'Yes, but mine are the same, since they're the same people. . . .'

'Then make yours. . . .'

Bernardt sculpted two images of women, placing them face to face with Helga's. But his two images had a stance suggesting violence directed at him. In spite of this, Bernardt said:

'You see? They're the same. . . . '

'Do you think so?'

After a pause, he went on:

'They are the same. The problem is that Helga hasn't told the truth. That's why they seem different.'

Clearly Helga was of the opposite opinion.

It is in just such cases that the use of this technique can succeed: when one person 'sees' – aesthetically – what the other thinks.

One can also ask the spect-actors to make their own image and then improvise the scene several times.

3 THE EXTRAVERSION TECHNIQUES

1 Improvisations

'STOP AND THINK'

This technique is based on the fact that while we can think at the speed of light we can only verbalise our thoughts at the speed of a horse-drawn cart.

Everything that is conscious is or can be verbalised. But, in the very time this verbalisation – this expression of our thoughts, emotions or sensations in words – is taking place, in the time it takes us give voice to, to articulate these words, our brains continue to produce thoughts. And, however fast we verbalise, new thoughts arise, thoughts that remain unverbalised.

This technique allows us – theatrically, aesthetically – to 'fix the moment' and to verify all the thoughts, layer upon layer, that are active at any given moment.

Stage one: the 'for the deaf' mode

The actors participating in the scene must present it in the 'for the deaf' mode, that is, magnifying each gesture. By trying to express themselves – without using words – in a manner which is so clear that even a deaf audience could understand them, or intuit what they mean, the actors awaken and activate other ideas, other sensations and emotions within themselves.

The other participants in the group observe this improvisation.

Stage two: the normal mode

The actors reimprovise the scene, reproducing, if possible, the gestures and movements – the visual language – of the first improvisation, but this time adding words to it. From this stage on, they will be able to perceive the disparities, the incongruities, between what they are doing and what they say they are intending to do.

Stage three: stop and think!

From time to time, the director will say: 'Stop!' He must carefully choose when to do it – moments he suspects to be richer in hidden thoughts than in thoughts revealed in the dialogue: the moments of 'suspense' or of 'crisis', the moments of doubt or tension.

When the director says: 'Stop! Think!', the actors freeze in mid-gesture and, without any other movement, without trying to complement each other, they must say everything that comes into their heads, without censorship or self-censorship. Absolutely anything that comes out will do, even – especially – things that contradict what they were expressing in their dialogue.

The actors should in no way seek coherence; the exercise is specifically designed to seek out the internal truth of each person, the hidden truth, the unformulated, the things which have not been put into words at the point of action. With the action suspended, we can see revealed the thoughts that were hidden therein, thoughts which have a much more vigorous and determinative effect on the action than those verbalised.

Normally, at the start, the actors have a tendency to reproduce the thoughts contained in the dialogue, with minor variations or in slightly different forms. It is up to the director to ensure that things do not stay like this and to urge the actors to throw themselves into the adventure: the exercise is about engendering the free association of thoughts, memories, images, sensations, emotions. Down with coherence!

Thus the action is punctuated with interruptions, with 'Stop! Think!' or 'Continue!' allowing an exploration of the subjacent (that which lies beneath the surface).

Stage four: the exchange of ideas

The director coordinates an exchange of ideas between all the participants. The goal of this exchange is to prepare the ground for the next stage. It is a good idea to discuss all the thoughts revealed in the exercise which we think might usefully be reiterated. Which thoughts should be replaced? What other thoughts should they be replaced by? And, most importantly, why? We believe – and this is only a hypothesis – that a clearly formulated and reiterated thought can stimulate the wish or will to which it corresponds. For instance, if I want something to succeed but continually think that it won't, it is obvious that I am not preparing myself for the thing I desire; I would even go so far as to say that, in such a case, deep down, I want my expressed wish for success to be unsuccessful.

Stage five: the reimprovisation with artificial pause

The actors improvise the scene over again, but this time, like the director in the previous section, the protagonist has the right to interrupt the action and, by means of an *artificial pause*, to express out loud all the thoughts which correspond to his 'declared wish'. If he wants to win the battle, he cannot think that he is going to lose it, come what may. Obviously, just thinking he will succeed is no guarantee of success, but dwelling on defeat is, effectively, a 'half-way' house on the way to that defeat, a preparation for defeat.

Stage six: the discussion

The director coordinates a discussion between all the participants.

THE PRACTICE

Gutman's revenge

In Rio, in June 1989, Gutman, the director of a theatre group, told us the following story. The actors in his group wanted to do nothing but act, an impossible ambition in a popular theatre group, where, of necessity, everybody must do everything – everyone must simultaneously be artist, technician, stagehand, whatever. As the actors shunned offstage work, it all fell back on Gutman, who felt he had to run the box office, clean the seats, build the sets, send out the press releases, etc. He had tried everything to convince them to share out the jobs that had to be done. The actors would say yes, he was right, but in practice, nothing changed.

Up until the day of the last straw . . . . Gutman, beside himself, decided to pull the production, in spite of the faithful public which was filling the theatre every day. Having taken the decision, Gutman announced it on a notice posted in the dressing rooms.

The scene went like this:

1 Gutman, on his own, was cleaning the chairs, organising the show.
2 Gutman informed a couple of the actors of his decision; the two of them protested, tried to dissuade him, but ended up convinced that there was no other solution.
3 A prima donna actress entered, the three of them informed her of the decision and left, leaving her alone in tears.

In the first stage, the *for the deaf* mode, in all that he did, to us Gutman seemed extremely vigorous. The pair of actors arrived, and, rather than fighting against the closure, they seemed to attack him. As soon as the prima donna actress came in, all three seemed to gang up against her.

In the second stage, the *normal* mode, nothing surprising happened. They had more or less the same dialogue as was recounted by Gutman at the start of the technique.

Then came the third stage, the *'Stop and think!'* stage. At the very beginning, when Gutman was still on his own, I stopped him three or four times midway through his physical activity of cleaning the seats and organising the show. All Gutman's thoughts were thoughts of revenge. He experienced pleasure at the thought of the suffering of the actors in the group when they discovered that he was pulling a show for which an audience existed. His thoughts were only of vengeance, of punishment.

In describing the scene, Gutman spoke to us of his great desire to continue the show, but under different conditions. He wanted to convince his colleagues to work, and he did not want to quit — he wanted to continue. However, in the *stop and think!* mode, after the entry of the pair of actors, every time I interrupted the action, without exception, Gutman gave vent to thoughts on the pleasure of vengeance. At no point did he have any thought of 'threatening', of issuing ultimata along the lines of 'either you start working or I stop the show'. All his thoughts were irreversible. He was doing his utmost to see the whole thing go up in smoke.

In the exchange of ideas which followed the 'stop and think!', Gutman realised that, in truth, even before the scene had started (in our theatre but also in reality) he had ceased to work with his colleagues. He had decided in advance that the only solution was to stop. To all appearances, he was still saying, 'The way things are going, you are forcing me to stop the show' but, in reality, he was saying, 'You lot forced me, and that is why I am punishing you.'

The leading actress was simply a scapegoat: everyone ganged up on her and took pleasure in her suffering.

Gutman concluded:

> 'It's true. If I had really wanted to go on, doubtless I would have threatened to stop the show. But, when I spoke to them, it wasn't a threat any more, it was a *fait accompli.*'

Soledad

In Rio, in June 1989, Soledad improvised a scene in which she was going to the tenant of the flat above hers to complain about a leak. The water from her neighbour's flat was running down Soledad's walls. She wanted him to mend his plumbing. The neighbour chatted very amiably about anything and everything, the weather, Soledad's spiritual aura, a visit he had made to Nepal, and, finally, he ended up selling her a book he had written. Soledad went away convinced that he wouldn't do anything about the water, and convinced that she would never read his book. A useless meeting, in which Soledad came across as a spectator, without the real will to get what she wanted. She allowed the neighbour to fob her off and went back to her place thwarted.[note]

We used the *stop and think!* mode. The neighbour's thoughts were more or less predictable. As for Soledad, before she had even knocked on the door, before she had even gone in, she was rehearsing phrases along the lines of, 'I know he won't do anything about it', 'I know that there is no point in going and talking to him', 'I know that it's no use trying.' This meant that the scene had barely started before it was over. What we were witnessing was not the conflict between Soledad and her neighbour. In reality, this scene was a mere epilogue. The real conflict was between the Soledad who wanted the plumbing mended and the Soledad who didn't believe she was worthy of this repair. The defeat – since Soledad did experience this event as a defeat – was taking place inside Soledad herself. The scene presented to us was a post-scene.

In both her scenes, Soledad had showed herself as apathetic, gentle, delicate, likeable. Some time later, in a different session, we did the game of the Opposite of Oneself (see p. 183). In this game, each person writes down a characteristic which she believes is non-existent in her personality and which she would like to

[note] The same thing had happened a few weeks before, with this same Soledad, when we used the rainbow of desire technique: the scene between her and her husband, who wouldn't hand over her records. In that scene too she was virtually passive (see p. 157 ff.).

experience by means of improvisation. After the improvisation, the observing participants must try to pin down what seemed different in each actor. At the end, we compare what the actor wrote on the piece of paper with what the observers said about them. Soledad wrote: 'I want to try to be delicate, likeable, gentle.' We improvised. At the end, I asked the participants what they had seen in each actor. Everyone was unanimous about Soledad:

'She behaved exactly like she always does.'

Always amiable, gentle, delicate, Soledad nevertheless thought of herself as violent and aggressive. Where was this violence, this aggression, located? Clearly inside the Soledad struggling against herself, stopping herself from externalising the aggression and the violence. While she wanted to be likeable, in fact she wanted to be likeable to herself, that is, to allow herself to be violent with her oppressors.

Some weeks later, I re-used, again with Soledad and working on a similar scene, the 'stop and think!' technique. This time I asked her to have only thoughts of the 'I want to because I want to' variety.

It was very curious: Soledad had no difficulty in being aggressive, violent, forceful. She even took pleasure in it. When I made this observation, her response was:

'I don't want people to think I'm like that. I'm not like that. I'm the way I showed before.'

'OK, a meek and mild person, but someone who can also be violent, aggressive. . . . Which of the two are you?'

Soledad laughed, and thought out loud:

'Both. . . .'

The meek and mild Soledad could usefully be tempered by the violent and aggressive Soledad, since, on its own, the first Soledad, the Soledad 'how she always is', would not be up to winning over either husband or neighbour. If, inside, she had them both, why not combine them in a more effective way?

THE ANALYTICAL REHEARSAL OF MOTIVATION

A single scene is improvised as many times as the number of 'pure emotions' that one can detect in it. For example: a single scene from *Romeo and Juliet* can be improvised with: (1) love; (2) hate; (3) fear. In each improvisation, the actors must concentrate solely on the emotion being analysed at that particular moment. When dealing with a written play, with a predetermined text, the actors cannot change the lines. If they do an improvisation with hate, and the text says 'I love you', the text will say that but with the emotion corresponding to the analytical rehearsal.

Having done as many improvisations as there are 'pure emotions' in the scene, we can try to improvise it one last time, this time aiming for a synthesis, that is, a mixture of all these emotions in what we call the 'dominants' of each character.[◉]

◉ See *Games for Actors and Non-Actors*, pp. 57–8 for a more extensive explanation of 'dominants'.

THE ANALYTICAL REHEARSAL OF STYLE

As for the preceding technique, the same scene is rehearsed in different styles. Sometimes, by changing the 'style' of the real-life scene, we can discover essential elements which this style was hiding.

Usually, we use extreme styles, for instance the clown or the 'psychological drama'. We can of course use the style which seems most appropriate, but we should try, however, at least once, to use the style furthest away from that of the real scene. The whole gamut of styles is open to us, and we can use them all: the western, the operatic, the musical comedy, the drama or the tragedy, all the styles and genres of theatre.

One can also imagine, instead of a style of genre, the style of a particular actor: 'What if all the characters were Charlie Chaplin?'; or the style of a particular director: 'What if all the characters came out of a Bergman film?'

THE PRACTICE

In Rio de Janeiro, in June 1989, Pedro told us a true story. Pedro is a musician, and once, in company with other striking musicians he went to picket the offices of their record company to protest about the very low wages the company gave them – wages which, to compound the offence, were only paid after unacceptable delays. With the help of a megaphone, they explained the facts to anyone willing to listen. Suddenly, a man comes out and says to the people outside that he has just paid the company for four hours of recording time, but is lacking a *cuica*◉ player, and he asks those present if there is a player among them ready to do this recording session. They refuse, since they are on strike. The man argues that he cannot afford to lose the money already committed; the strikers argue that their strike will be of benefit to everyone, in the long run. The temperature rises, tempers fray, the man gets a revolver out of his pocket and the musicians flee, scared out of their wits.

The improvisation of the scene left us absolutely horrified at the attitude of the man with the revolver.

We proposed, first of all, the 'Mexican drama'◉ style. And we split our sides laughing. The man with the revolver in this version became a less threatening figure, the terror of the gun was pushed into the background and he now became, in our eyes, the *cuica* man. And when he tearfully sobbed that his life depended on a *cuica*, a comical thing for one's life to depend on, he forced us to see the ridiculousness of the situation.

Then we suggested the style of 'psychological drama taken seriously'. In this version many things came to light which were not visible in the original scene. On the part of the man – who was back to being the man with the revolver – genuine anxieties became apparent which the comic nature of the *cuica* had concealed. In fact, he was just a poor composer, putting all his money into the recording of a track which, in his dreams, was going to make him famous. He was jeopardising a career which in his imagination would be full of glory and money. He saw it threatened by the absence of a *cuica*. This man's problem was immediate, concrete, visible.

None of the musicians' reasons appeared to us to be any less important: they were full of good sense. But what came to the fore was their intransigence, their refusal of dialogue. At no point did they seek to discover what was going on with this man, at no point did they try to find possible solutions to his problem. They simply reiterated the same truths in the form of 'slogans', and to the man's immediate need their only response was the promise of future benefits for the whole corporation. But the man needed the *cuica* now, and not in the future.

◉ A percussion instrument which resembles a small drum, but which has a wooden stick inside, protruding from the middle of the skin. The *cuica* player rubs this wooden stick with a damp cloth, touching the skin on the other side with his other hand, thus emitting a curious wailing sound. In Brazil they say that the *cuica* cries (A.J.).

◉ A very popular soap opera form, usually involving tears, suffering and tragedy, redeemed by pure love, eternal goodness, etc. (A.B.).

The musicians' just causes turned into 'slogans', into abstract demagogy.

BREAKING THE OPPRESSION

This technique, already described in my preceding books, essentially consists of improvising the same scene three times:

1 as it happened in real life;
2 trying, in the improvisation, to bring about the result desired but unrealised in reality;
3 swapping roles bewteen protagonist and antagonist.

ACTION! WE'RE SHOOTING

1 The scene is improvised the way it happened in real life.
2 The scene is improvised a second time. This time, however, the director interrupts whenever she feels any point needs clarification; in order to attract the protagonist's attention to a particular detail which she thinks is important; to make the protagonist aware of something that he is doing without realising; finally, to verify if the protagonist has alternatives to the situation which he himself has offered up.
3 After working on the specific point, the director says, like a film director: 'Action! We're shooting!' and the actors reimprovise the scene as many times and with as many interruptions as necessary for its complete clarification.

SOMATISATION

After a first improvisation, the actors reimprovise the scene trying to physically exaggerate their emotions and sensations: fear becomes actual shivering, wanting to run away, vomiting, cold in the pit of the stomach, and so on.

2 Games

THE EMBASSY BALL

This game is based on a real event, which happened in Brasilia during the time of the armed struggle against the dictatorship.

The actors invent characters, who can be imaginary or real – princes, magnates, ambassadors, papal nuncios, etc. All are gathered at the Foreign Office, which is giving them a reception.

In the first part of this game, each actor plays her character arriving and circulating at this official function. After a few minutes, the waiter – one actor must play the part of a waiter – serves up a chocolate cake which supposedly contains a strong dose of marijuana (this really happened in Brasilia in 1971). From this moment on, the actors must enact a struggle between two characters: the one being the character they have chosen, sober, and the other being that character out of control, as revealed by the fictive hallucinogenic dose. They must endeavour not to completely eliminate the former, in order to show the struggle between the two.

Finally, the effects of the drug having worn off, the first characters are in charge once again and the improvisation finishes as if nothing had happened.

THE OPPOSITE OF ONESELF

The group is divided in two. Each actor in the first group writes on a piece of paper her name and the type of opposite personality that she would like to try out: the calm person who would like to be highly strung, the timid person who wants to be courageous, or vice versa. Anything goes – whatever each person would really like to be or would like to try out in order to discover how it would feel if she really was like that.

Over a few minutes, the actors improvise with this new personality. Within that time, the director should ask them to return to normal at least once, but then, immediately afterwards, to resume the experimental character.

At the end, the observers of the second group must say what differences they noticed between the improvised and normal characters of each person. The participants' observations are then compared with what the actors wrote on their pieces of paper.

AWAKENING DORMANT CHARACTERS

This technique is similar to the preceding one, with the slight difference that this time it is the participant-observers who must suggest the characteristics to be improvised by the actors.

In this kind of game the actors who are playing sometimes do not share the same mental picture of the place they are in and they imagine different givens. This means that the improvisation may be happening in a variety of different spaces and that the relations between characters may be differently understood by each actor, who may also project, on to each of the others, characteristics different from those that these other characters have attributed to themselves. This apparent surrealism should not be taken as an obstacle to the improvisation. On the contrary, it should be taken for granted.

3 Shows

The Forum Theatre and Invisible Theatre forms, which were explained at length, demonstrated and illustrated in my previous books, can be – and are – extremely useful as extraversion work for a protagonist who wants to try alternatives to her usual behaviour.

FORUM THEATRE

Forum Theatre consists, in essence, of proposing to a group of spectators, after a first improvisation of a scene, that they replace the protagonist and try to improvise variations on his actions. The real protagonist should, ultimately, improvise the variation that has motivated him the most.

INVISIBLE THEATRE

Invisible Theatre consists of rehearsing a scene with actions that the protagonist would like to try out in real life, and improvising it in a place where these events could really happen and in front of an audience who, unaware that they are an audience, accordingly act as if the improvised scene was real. Thus, the improvised scene becomes reality. Fiction penetrates reality. What the protagonist had rehearsed as a plan, a blueprint, now becomes an act.

The real goal of the arsenal of the Theatre of the Oppressed is to contribute to the preparation of the future rather than waiting for it to happen.

POSTSCRIPT: THE TECHNIQUES AND OURSELVES: AN EXPERIMENT IN INDIA

This book was already with the publishers when I went to Calcutta in India (February–March 1994), at the invitation of Jana Sanskriti, a group which develops popular theatre and educational methods among peasants, to work with forty theatre people from all over West Bengal, Bangladesh and Pakistan. During my work there it became evident once again that techniques – such as those described in this book – need to be adapted to be useful to the people who practise them, rather than vice versa.

This was my first visit to India: the culture shock was inevitably extreme. I was especially sensitive to the traffic jams. In most cities, priority is usually given to the vehicle coming from the left, or from the right; in Rio, priority is given to the heaviest vehicle, wherever it is coming from. In Calcutta, it seemed to me that it is given to the vehicle with the most unpleasant horn sound! And everyone seems to blow their horns, all the time.

Besides the tremendous acoustic and air pollution, the streets are full of pot-holes and craters, so the drivers are forced to zigzag to avoid them; drivers already preoccupied with avoiding pedestrians, bicycles, tricycles, rickshaws (all, whether motorised or cycle-driven, driven by shoeless men), and, last but not least, the cows. I was amazed at the sight of so many sacred cows wandering around without interference. I asked a journalist whether we were allowed to persuade the cows to get out of the road if they were obstructing traffic, as I had often seen them doing. She answered: 'Politely, yes!'

Husbands don't seem to be so polite to their wives. I asked the group to improvise a common, everyday scene of a couple at home. The husband shouted at his wife, protesting about her father's lateness in paying the instalments on her promised dowry. Eventually, the husband ended up killing the woman, burning the corpse before burying it, and preparing to marry again, this time for a dowry to be paid in cash, before the marriage.

The discussion amongst the participants centred on whether this was a common, everyday scene, or something that happened only occasionally. Some thought it not so frequent, but no one considered it to be an exceptional event, especially in the countryside.

From the very first exercises, I understood that I was facing people from a culture very different from those with which I was used to working in Europe, Africa and the three Americas. For instance, when we were doing the Image of the Hour, at a certain point I said, 'Show the moment you wake up on your birthday.' The exercise came to a halt: no one knew the date of their birthday, and they didn't seem to mind.

Jana Sanskriti had asked me to introduce them to the intro-spective techniques. This was the first time I had used these techniques with a group entirely made up of peasants and people who work with peasants; very poor peasants, since most of them earn only the minimum wage for peasants in India – one dollar a day – and this only for three to six months of the year.

We did lots of games and image techniques during the first two days. On the third day, I decided to use the Rainbow of Desire. A very timid girl offered the story of her own marriage for 'the rainbow'. She was trembling, but, even so, was able to improvise the domestic violence and afterwards to create some images of her desires.

The first was an image of her strangling herself – as though her desire was to accomplish her husband's desire. The second, her leaving the house – without doubt again her husband's desire. Then an image of her talking to him; her trying to seduce him, stretching a leg across his stomach (the actor playing the husband immediately pulled away from her!); finally, her trying to kill him.

I was happy to see that timid girl's courage in making concrete images of her desires, happy also to see the resonance of her images amongst the participants, especially amongst the women who jumped on stage to replace her in her images. When she finished, I felt that her strongest desire at that moment did not concern her husband at all: she had proposed herself as a protag-onist, when her feelings were hidden even from herself, but there and then, seeing her desires take concrete physical form, she felt ashamed of revealing them to the others, and to herself. Her desire was to stop the whole thing.

Following the sequence of steps in the Rainbow of Desire, she would have fought or stimulated her desires, one by one, in the stage where the conscious will confronts the unconscious desires. But I became aware that she was weeping – she did not wish to, or could not, continue. So I bypassed that step and went directly to the agora of desires, in which each desire fights its extreme opposite. The girl went back to the audience to see how her desires, which reflected the desires of most of the women there, would fight each other on stage, as they were fighting deep in her heart.

On the last day of this short workshop, we started with 'The Two Revelations of St Teresa'.[⊚] In pairs (parent–child), the actors improvise a common situation, during which each makes a revelation to the other, for better or worse. Ninety per cent of the revelations made by the women dealt with sex and repression: most revealed that they were in love and wanted to marry a man from a lower caste; or, if the man belonged to the same caste as them or a higher caste, they wanted to choose their own partner rather than passively accept their father's choice. Such revelations were enough to completely explode, to shatter, their relationship with the father, a relationship based on absolute submission. All the women wanted was to be able to choose for themselves whom they married – they didn't even dare talk about free love.

⊚ See Games for Actors and Non-Actors, London: Routledge, 1992, p. 159.

After this we worked on the Analytical Image, and once again the life of the couple was the theme chosen. Bearing in mind what had happened the day before, I did not ask any woman to expose herself or tell her own real-life story. I decided to ask them to 'invent' a typical possible situation. And I asked them to improvise using as models people they knew well, not themselves. Of course, since they were not enacting their 'real story', they felt free and safe to play their real emotions, feelings and thoughts. They had not stated 'This is me', so they felt protected, free to show themselves as they really were.

To make them even more at ease, I asked men to make images of women and vice versa; thus each party could show and see their critiques of the other.

This was not the normal way to use these techniques, but the techniques were invented to be useful to people and, as I have stressed, not with the goal of adapting the people to suit the techniques. They were made for human beings, not human beings for them.

In the Theatre of the Oppressed, the Oppressed are the Subject – Theatre is their language.